Applying Evidence-Based Concepts in the Treatment of Distal Radius Fractures in the 21st Century

Editor

KEVIN C. CHUNG

HAND CLINICS

www.hand.theclinics.com

Consulting Editor
KEVIN C. CHUNG

May 2021 • Volume 37 • Number 2

ELSEVIER

1600 John F. Kennedy Boulevard • Suite 1800 • Philadelphia, Pennsylvania, 19103-2899

http://www.theclinics.com

HAND CLINICS Volume 37, Number 2
May 2021 ISSN 0749-0712, ISBN-13: 978-0-323-83612-8

Editor: Lauren Boyle
Developmental Editor: Arlene B. Campos

Hand Clinics (ISSN 0749-0712) is published quarterly by Elsevier Inc., 360 Park Avenue South, New York, NY 10010-1710. Months of publication are February, May, August, and November. Business and Editorial Offices: 1600 John F. Kennedy Blvd., Ste. 1800, Philadelphia, PA 19103-2899. Customer Service Office: 3251 Riverport Lane, Maryland Heights, MO 63043. Periodicals postage paid at New York, NY and at additional mailing offices. Subscription price is $439.00 per year (domestic individuals), $1039.00 per year (domestic institutions), $100.00 per year (domestic students/residents), $501.00 per year (Canadian individuals), $1086.00 per year (Canadian institutions), $562.00 per year (international individuals), $1086.00 per year (international institutions), $256.00 (international students/residents), and $100.00 (Canadian students/residents). Foreign air speed delivery is included in all *Clinics* subscription prices. All prices are subject to change without notice. **POSTMASTER:** Send address changes to *Hand Clinics*, Elsevier Health Sciences Division, Subscription Customer Service, 3251 Riverport Lane, Maryland Heights, MO 63043. Customer Service (orders, claims, online, change of address): Elsevier Health Sciences Division, Subscription **Customer Service, 3251 Riverport Lane, Maryland Heights, MO 63043. Tel: 1-800-654-2452 (U.S. and Canada); 314-447-8871 (outside U.S. and Canada). Fax: 314-447-8029. E-mail: journalscustomerservice-usa@elsevier.com (for print support); journalsonlinesupport-usa@elsevier.com (for online support).**

Reprints. For copies of 100 or more of articles in this publication, please contact the Commercial Reprints Department, Elsevier Inc., 360 Park Avenue South, New York, New York 10010-1710. Tel.: 212-633-3874; Fax: 212-633-3820; E-mail: reprints@elsevier.com.

Hand Clinics is covered in *MEDLINE/PubMed (Index Medicus), Current Contents/Clinical Medicine, EMBASE/Excerpta Medica,* and *ISI/BIOMED.*

Contributors

CONSULTING EDITOR

KEVIN C. CHUNG, MD, MS
Charles B. G. de Nancrede Professor of
Surgery, Professor of Plastic Surgery and
Orthopaedic Surgery, Chief of Hand Surgery,
Michigan Medicine, The University of Michigan
Health System, University of Michigan
Comprehensive Hand Center, Assistant Dean
for Faculty Affairs, Associate Director of Global
REACH, University of Michigan Medical
School, Ann Arbor, Michigan, USA

EDITOR

KEVIN C. CHUNG, MD, MS
Charles B. G. de Nancrede Professor of
Surgery, Professor of Plastic Surgery and
Orthopaedic Surgery, Chief of Hand Surgery,
Michigan Medicine, The University of Michigan
Health System, University of Michigan
Comprehensive Hand Center, Assistant Dean
for Faculty Affairs, Associate Director of Global
REACH, University of Michigan Medical
School, Ann Arbor, Michigan, USA

AUTHORS

ASHLEY B. ANDERSON, MD
Department of Orthopaedic Surgery, Walter
Reed National Military Medical Center,
Bethesda, Maryland, USA

ETHAN BLACKBURN, MD
Norton Healthcare, Hand and Upper Extremity
Surgery, Louisville Arm and Hand, Clinical
Instructor, University of Louisville, Orthopaedic
Surgery, Louisville, Kentucky, USA

DAVID J. BOZENTKA, MD
Doctor of Medicine, Chief of Hand Surgery,
Associate Professor, Department of
Orthopaedic Surgery, University of
Pennsylvania, Chief of Orthopaedic Surgery,
Penn Presbyterian Medical Center,
Philadelphia, Pennsylvania, USA

KEVIN C. CHUNG, MD, MS
Charles B. G. de Nancrede Professor of
Surgery, Professor of Plastic Surgery and
Orthopaedic Surgery, Chief of Hand Surgery,
Michigan Medicine, The University of Michigan
Health System, University of Michigan
Comprehensive Hand Center, Assistant Dean
for Faculty Affairs, Associate Director of Global
REACH, University of Michigan Medical
School, Ann Arbor, Michigan, USA

LAUREN KATE DUTTON, MD
Department of Orthopedic Surgery, Mayo
Clinic, Rochester, Minnesota, USA

CHRISTOPHER J. DY, MD, MPH
Assistant Professor, Department of
Orthopaedic Surgery, Washington University in
St. Louis, St Louis, Missouri, USA

LAUREN FADER, MD
Department of Orthopaedic Surgery, University
of Louisville, Louisville, Kentucky, USA

NATHANIEL FOGEL, MD
Department of Orthopaedic Surgery, Stanford
University Medical Center, Redwood City,
California, USA

CHRISTOPHER J. GOT, MD
Member of ASSH and AOA, Assistant
Professor, Department of Orthopedics, Brown
University, University Orthopedics Inc,
Lifespan Rhode Island Hospital, Miriam
Hospital, Providence, Rhode Island, USA

MICHAEL B. GOTTSCHALK, MD
Associate Professor, Department of
Orthopaedics, Adjunct Associate Professor,
Division of Plastic Surgery, Director of Clinical
Research, Upper Extremity Division Director,
Hand and Upper Extremity Fellowship Director,
Emory School of Medicine, Atlanta Veteran
Affairs Hospital, Grady Memorial Hospital,
Morehouse School of Medicine

DAVID W. GRANT, MD, MASc
Hand Fellow, University of Michigan Medical
School, The University of Michigan Health
System, University of Michigan
Comprehensive Hand Center, Ann Arbor,
Michigan, USA

RUBY GREWAL, MD, MSc, FRCSC
Professor, Division of Orthopaedic Surgery,
Roth|McFarlane Hand and Upper Limb Center,
Western University, London, Ontario, Canada

MATTHEW J. HALL, MD
Harvard Combined Orthopaedic Residency
Program, Boston, Massachusetts, USA

ASIF M. ILYAS, MD, MBA
The Rothman Orthopaedic Institute, Thomas
Jefferson University, Rothman Institute,
Philadelphia, Pennsylvania, USA

PAUL M. INCLAN, MD
Resident Physician, Department of
Orthopaedic Surgery, Washington University in
St. Louis, St Louis, Missouri, USA

PAUL KOONER, MD
Orthopaedic Surgery PGY1, McGill University,
Montreal, Quebec, Canada

CHRISTINA NYPAVER, MD
Doctor of Medicine, Resident Physician,
Department of Orthopaedic Surgery, University
of Pennsylvania, Philadelphia, Pennsylvania,
USA

PETER J. OSTERGAARD, MD
Harvard Combined Orthopaedic Residency
Program, Boston, Massachusetts, USA

NICHOLAS PULOS, MD
Assistant Professor, Department of Orthopedic
Surgery, Mayo Clinic, Rochester, Minnesota,
USA

JEREMY E. RADUCHA, MD
Orthopedic Resident, Department of
Orthopedics, Brown University, Lifespan Inc,
Rhode Island Hospital, Miriam Hospital,
Providence, Rhode Island, USA

PETER CHARLES RHEE, DO, MS
Associate Professor, Department of
Orthopedic Surgery, Mayo Clinic, Rochester,
Minnesota, USA

TAMARA D. ROZENTAL, MD
Chief, Division of Hand and Upper Extremity
Surgery, Department of Orthopedics, Beth
Israel Deaconess Medical Center, Professor,
Harvard Medical School, Boston,
Massachusetts, USA

LILI E. SCHINDELAR, MD, MPH
The Rothman Orthopaedic Institute, Thomas
Jefferson University, Rothman Institute,
Philadelphia, Pennsylvania, USA

ALEXANDER Y. SHIN, MD
Professor, Department of Orthopedic Surgery,
Mayo Clinic, Rochester, Minnesota, USA

SCOTT M. TINTLE, MD, CDR MC USN
Chief Hand Surgery, Fellowship Director,
Associate Professor of Surgery, Department of
Orthopaedic Surgery, Walter Reed National

Military Medical Center, Bethesda, Maryland, USA

ERIC R. WAGNER, MD, MS
Assistant Professor, Department of Orthopaedics, Adjunct Assistant Professor, Division of Plastic Surgery, Director of Research, Upper Extremity Division Director, Emory School of Medicine, Grady Memorial Hospital, Morehouse School of Medicine, Emory Orthopaedics and Spine Center, Atlanta, Georgia, USA

JEFFREY YAO, MD
Professor, Department of Orthopaedic Surgery, Stanford University Medical Center, Redwood City, California, USA

Contents

This article reviews the impact of the most cited works on distal radius fractures. Judged by the most cited works in this field, distal radius fracture research has followed other paradigm shifts in the history of science. Landmark papers showed that restoring premorbid anatomy led to better outcomes, and a plurality of fixation strategies emerged. A breakthrough in technology came with volar plating, and the new paradigm emerged: precise anatomic reduction is achieved typically with volar plates, unless fragment-specific approaches are needed. This paradigm is being challenged as the association among malunion, arthritis, and function continues to be understood. The best treatment of distal radius fractures in the elderly has also evolved through time.

Distal radius fractures, like many articular and periarticular fractures, can make it difficult to determine the true number, location, and orientation of fracture fragments. This article should help the reader work through imaging interpretation starting from the initial, often displaced radiographs to postreduction imaging and determination if further 3-dimensional imaging is necessary.

Operative intervention for distal radius fractures is typically reserved for patients with displaced fractures that may result in bothersome compromises in function, although patient-specific factors (age, activity level, and preference) are considered. Operative intervention is associated with earlier improvement in function but exposes the patient to the risk of anesthesia and surgery. Although surgery is associated with an initial increase in cost of care, the benefits of earlier return to activity may offset these increases. Efforts to contain cost through implant selection, use of ambulatory surgical centers, and judicious referrals for postoperative therapy can aid surgeons in delivering high-value care.

Distal radius fractures (DRFs) are among the most common upper extremity injuries. Multiple medical conditions now are evaluated by standardized outcome sets that enable comparability. Recent international working groups have provided consensus statements for outcomes measurement after DRFs. These statements emphasized the growing importance of patient-reported outcome measures as well as traditional measures, including pain assessment, radiographic alignment, performance, and assessment of complications. A standardized instrument and timeline for measuring outcomes following DRFs offers clinicians, researchers, and health care economists a powerful tool. This article reviews the current evidence and provides recommendations for a DRF standardized outcome set.

Distal radius fractures are common in the elderly population, second only to hip fractures in frequency. Historically, these injuries were treated almost exclusively without surgery, but an increase in operative management has occurred with development of volar locked plating in the early 2000s. Functional outcomes are similar between conservative and surgical treatment, but most studies assume low functional demands in older patients. Many elderly individuals today are active and independent. Decision-making in this higher-demand population is difficult. This article provides current evidence to facilitate informed, individualized decision-making when treating distal radius fractures in geriatric patients.

Distal radius fractures are one of the most common orthopedic injuries. After history, physical examination, and diagnostic imaging, treatment begins with closed reduction and immobilization to restore an upper extremity that has both acceptable alignment and stability. Whether for definitive nonoperative management or in preparation for surgical fixation, it is important to understand the principles of closed reduction and immobilization. This article presents a brief review of indications and a technical guide to successful closed reduction and casting for the orthopedic surgeon.

Distal radius fractures are the most common upper extremity fracture that present to US emergency departments. Given the variable presentation, including age and fracture pattern, there are many techniques that have been utilized to treat them. Closed reduction and percutaneous pin (CRPP) fixation remains a viable option in extra-articular and simple intra-articular fracture patterns. CRPP techniques flourished in the mid-twentieth century until the treatment patterns shifted to primarily volar-locked plating in the twenty-first century. Although several meta-analyses have been performed comparing outcomes and complications of CRPP versus alternative methods, controversy remains over which treatments are superior.

There are several options for plate fixation of distal radius fractures. Volar plating has broad applicability and consistent outcomes, and thus is the most commonly used plate type. Dorsal plates are advantageous for specific fracture patterns, and can provide direct fracture reduction and buttressing, but may be prominent and can cause tendon irritation. Bridge plates offer an alternative to external fixation while avoiding the complications with prominent hardware, because they span highly comminuted fractures and can be used for immediate weight bearing; however, they require plate removal. Choice of plate fixation should depend on fracture type, patient factors, and surgeon experience.

High-energy distal radius fractures frequently result in comminution with intra-articular fragmentation. Knowledge of predictable patterns of injury allows the surgeon to develop a preoperative plan for anatomic reduction and stable fixation of individual fragments that are too small or too distal to be fixed with standard volar locked plating. We review the column model, which organizes the distal radius into an intermediate column, radial column, and pedestal as the basis of a reconstructive algorithm and emphasize the importance of the volar ulnar fragment. Specific reduction and fixation techniques are described to assist the surgeon in treating these injuries.

Wrist arthroscopy in the setting of distal radius fractures allows for direct visualization of the articular surface and treatment of associated soft tissue injuries. Arthroscopic techniques may be used to fine tune reductions with residual articular step-off or gap after an initial reduction attempt and are critical for addressing free articular fragments and die-punch lesions. Surgeon training, experience, and comfort with wrist arthroscopy remains a barrier to widespread adoption of this technique. Level I studies are needed to investigate whether improved articular reduction leads to meaningful clinical differences.

In this article, we discuss the incidence and types of injuries to the distal radioulnar joint (DRUJ) that occur in the setting of a distal radius fracture. We review the anatomy of the distal radioulnar joint, which is critical to understanding its biomechanics, and how injury could cause symptomatic incongruency and instability. We highlight how patients with an injury to the distal radioulnar joint might present both at the time of injury and after treatment of a distal radius fracture, the appropriate workup, the available treatment options, and the evidence-based literature.

The role of hand therapy in management of distal radius fractures remains unclear. Some evidence demonstrates that initiating early range of motion and urging patients to return to routine activities of daily living as soon as possible may produce favorable outcomes that are as effective as formal supervised therapy. Extended supervised therapy does not appear to impact outcomes and a single instruction session with a home-based program produces similar results. Although we feel that formal structured therapy may have a role in select high-risk patients, the literature remains unclear on which patients would benefit most from formal supervised therapy.

Complex regional pain syndrome (CRPS) is a chronic pain condition characterized by a constellation of signs and symptoms including pain out of proportion to the injury or insult, autonomic dysfunction, trophic changes, and impaired function. CRPS may occur following either conservative or surgical management of distal radius fractures and can significantly complicate the trajectory of a patient's recovery. Although the incidence, diagnosis, prevention, and treatment of this condition have been extensively studied, optimal methods to identify, prevent, and treat this condition remain controversial. This article reviews the available literature on the diagnosis and treatment of CRPS in distal radius fractures.

HAND CLINICS

THE CLINICS ARE AVAILABLE ONLINE!
Access your subscription at:
www.theclinics.com

HAND CLINICS

Preface

The Contemporary View of Distal Radius Fracture Management

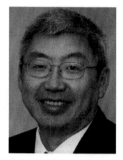

Kevin C. Chung, MD, MS
Editor

For more than 2 centuries, distal radius fracture has been a fascination for surgeons because of the complexity of this anatomic region and the controversies surrounding its treatment. With the application of patient-rated outcomes instruments, we have a greater understanding of the impact of the treatment decisions we make to optimize patient function, while considering the fracture patterns, patients' socioeconomic status, and most importantly, their wishes and autonomy. Although spirited discussions when reviewing radiographs lead to intricate treatments options, the data from the WRIST trial highlight the importance of patient-centered care by tailoring the treatment based not only on the fracture patterns but also on a shared decision-making process to optimize outcomes by considering the patients' needs.

This issue of *Hand Clinics* invites an expansive discussion on the surgical but also nonsurgical treatments of distal radius fractures. Rather than treating every patient with internal fixation, we realized that surgeons must be equipped with all the surgical and nonsurgical options, while also considering the rate of recovery and the cost associated with the treatment. I am grateful to the authors of this issue, who are noted authorities in managing this injury, for their sage guidance, introducing a new era in the treatment of this vexing injury. Similarly, I appreciate the readership of *Hand Clinics*, that strives to provide the most up-to-date data to inform current practice. I am privileged to learn along with you as Editor-in-Chief on various fascinating topics that shape this specialty. Thank you for your support, and best wishes on your care of your patients.

Kevin C. Chung, MD, MS
Comprehensive Hand Center
Michigan Medicine
Ann Arbor, MI 48105, USA

E-mail address:
kecchung@med.umich.edu

Hand Clin 37 (2021) xiii
https://doi.org/10.1016/j.hcl.2021.03.001
0749-0712/21/© 2021 Published by Elsevier Inc.

A Critical Assessment of the Most Cited Papers on Distal Radius Fractures

David W. Grant, MD, MASc[a,b], Kevin C. Chung, MD, MS[b,c],*

KEYWORDS

• Distal radius fractures • Citation analysis • Surgery evolution

KEY POINTS

• Bacorn and Kurtzke demonstrated that distal radius fractures led to greater morbidity than appreciated in the early half of the last century and suggested better methods were needed to treat them.
• Gartland and Werley, and Knirk and Jupiter showed that restoring anatomy correlated with less wrist arthritis after the injury. The significance of this association is still being understood, but their findings guide clinical treatment today.
• The application of the volar locking system by Orbay and Fernandez changed the management of distal radius fracture because the rigidity provided by this approach yields better outcomes owing to earlier return of function.
• Treatment of distal radius fractures in the elderly has alternated between operative and nonoperative strategies, with new studies clarifying patient factors as more important than age.

INTRODUCTION

Citation analyses repeatedly find articles on distal radius fracture (DRF) as some of the most cited articles in wrist surgery and hand surgery ever published.[1–3] The most cited articles include Phalen's series on carpal tunnel syndrome,[4] Napier's reporting of basic prehensile hand movements,[5] and the landmark DRF articles by Gartland and Werley,[6] and Knirk and Jupiter.[7] In article, the authors review the most cited articles and put them into context to understand their impact on DRF research and clinical practice.

The authors used several previously published citation analyses of hand surgery with different methodologies to capture important articles in their field.[1–3] They extracted all references of articles on DRFs, produced a list of the top 35 most cited articles in DRFs included in these citation analyses, and placed them into thematic groups (**Box 1**).

Citation analysis is just one way of understanding the evolution of research on DRFs. Citation frequency is often used but is not easy to interpret. Productive researchers may cite their own work, making a highly cited article reflective of the authors' productivity rather than the article's wider importance. In addition, a highly cited article is not necessarily a high-quality article. Indeed, most articles in this group are not representations

Financial Disclosure: Dr K.C. Chung receives funding from the National Institutes of Health and book royalties from Wolters Kluwer and Elsevier. He is a consultant for Axogen and Integra. The remaining author has nothing to disclose. No funding was received for this article.

[a] Fellow, Combined Hand Surgery Fellowship, University of Michigan, Ann Arbor, MI, USA; [b] Section of Plastic Surgery, The University of Michigan Health System, University of Michigan Comprehensive Hand Center, 1500 East Medical Center Drive, 2130 Taubman Center, SPC 5340, Ann Arbor, MI 48109-5340, USA; [c] Section of Plastic Surgery, Department of Surgery, University of Michigan Medical School, Ann Arbor, MI, USA

* Corresponding author. Section of Plastic Surgery, The University of Michigan Health System, University of Michigan Comprehensive Hand Center, 1500 East Medical Center Drive, 2130 Taubman Center, SPC 5340, Ann Arbor, MI 48109-5340.

E-mail address: kecchung@med.umich.edu

Hand Clin 37 (2021) 189–196
https://doi.org/10.1016/j.hcl.2021.02.001

hand.theclinics.com

Box 1
Most cited papers in distal radius fractures, grouped by theme

Theme 1: Anatomic alignment

- Gartland JJ, Werley CW. Evaluation of healed Colles fractures. J Bone Joint Surg Am. 1951; 33(4):895–907 - PMID: 14880544

- Bacorn RW, Kurtzke JF. Colles fracture—a study of 2000 cases from the New York State Workmen's Compensation Board. J Bone Joint Surg Am. 1953; 35(3):643–658 - PMID: 13069552

- Sarmiento A, Pratt GW, Berry NC et al. Colles fractures—functional bracing in supination. J Bone Joint Surg Am. 1975; 57(3):311 - PMID: 1123382

- Cooney WP, Linscheid RL, Dobyns JH. External pin fixation for unstable Colles fractures. J Bone Joint Surg Am. 1979; 61(6):840–845 - PMID: 479230

- Cooney WP, Dobyns JH, Linscheid RL. Complications of Colles fractures. J Bone Joint Surg Am. 1980; 62 (4):613–619 - PMID: 6155380

- Pogue, DJ, Viegas, SF, Patterson, RM, et al. Effects of distal radius fracture malunion on wrist joint mechanics. J Hand Surg Am. 1990;15(5):721–727 - PMID 2229966

- McQueen M, Caspers J. Colles fracture—does the anatomical result affect the final function? J Bone Joint Surg Br. 1988; 70(4):649–651 - PMID: 3403617

- Knirk JL, Jupiter JB. Intra-articular fractures of the distal end of the radius in young adults. J Bone Joint Surg Am. 1986; 68(5):647–659 - PMID: 3722221

- Trumble TE, Schmitt SR, Vedder NB. Factors affecting functional outcome of displaced intra-articular distal radius fractures. J Hand Surg Am. 1994; 19(2):325–340 - PMID: 8201203

- Bradway JK, Amadio PC, Cooney WP. Open reduction and internal fixation of displaced, comminuted intra-articular fractures of the distal end of the radius. J Bone Joint Surg Am. 1989; 71(6):839–847 - PMID: 2745480

- Catalano LW III, Cole RJ, Gelberman RH, Evanoff BA, Gilula LA, Borrelli J II. Displaced intra-articular fractures of the distal aspect of the radius—long-term results in young adults after open reduction and internal fixation. J Bone Joint Surg Am. 1997;79(9):1290–1302 - PMID 9314391

Theme 2: Hardware

- McQueen MM, Hajducka C, CourtBrown CM. Redisplaced unstable fractures of the distal, radius—a prospective randomised comparison of four methods of treatment. J Bone Joint Surg Br. 1996;78(3):404–409 - PMID 8636175

- Carter PR; Frederick HA; Laseter GF. Open reduction and internal fixation of unstable distal radius fractures with a low-profile plate: a multicenter study of 73 fractures. J Hand Surg Am. 1998 Mar;23(2):300-7 - PMID 9556273

- Ring D, Jupiter JB, Brennwald J, Büchler U, Hastings H II. Prospective multicenter trial of a plate for dorsal fixation of distal radius fractures. J Hand Surg Am. 1997 ;22(5):777–784 - PMID 9330133

- Jupiter JB, Winters S, Sigman S, et al. Repair of five distal radius fractures with an investigational cancellous bone cement: a preliminary report. J Orthop Trauma. 1997;11(2):110–106 - PMID 9057146

- Kambouroglou GK, Axelrod TS. Complications of the AO/ASIF titanium distal radius plate system (pi plate) in internal fixation of the distal radius: a brief report. J Hand Surg Am. 1998;23(4):737–741 - PMID 9708391

- Orbay JL, Fernandez DL. Volar fixation for dorsally displaced fractures of the distal radius: a preliminary report. J Hand Surg Am. 2002 Mar;27(2):205-15 - PMID 11901379

- Chung KC; Watt AJ; Kotsis SV, et al. Treatment of unstable distal radial fractures with the volar locking plating system. J Bone Joint Surg Am. 2006 Dec;88(12):2687-94

- Rozental TD, Blazar PE. Functional outcome and complications after volar plating for dorsally displaced, unstable fractures of the distal radius. J Hand Surg Am. 2006;31(3):359–365 - PMID 16516728

- Musgrave DS; Idler RS. Volar fixation of dorsally displaced distal radius fractures using the 2.4-mm locking compression plates. J Hand Surg Am. 2005 Jul;30(4):743-9

- Arora R, Lutz M, Hennerbichler A, Krappinger D, Espen D, Gabl M. Complications following internal fixation of unstable distal radius fracture with a palmar locking-plate. J Orthop Trauma. 2007;21(5):316–322 - PMID 17485996

- Rozental TD; Blazar PE; Franko OI; et al. Functional outcomes for unstable distal radial fractures treated with open reduction and internal fixation or closed reduction and percutaneous fixation a prospective randomized trial. J Bone Joint Surg Am. 2009 Aug;91(8):1837-46 - PMID 19651939

- Wright TW; Horodyski MB; Smith DW. Functional outcome of unstable distal radius fractures: ORIF with a volar fixed-angle tine plate versus external fixation. J Hand Surg Am. 2005 Mar;30(2):289-99 - PMID 15781351

- Egol K; Walsh M; Tejwani N; et al. Bridging external fixation and supplementary Kirschner-wire fixion versus volar locked plating for unstable fractures of the distal radius - a randomised, prospective trial. J Bone Joint Surg Br. 2008 Sep;90(9):1214-21

- Wei DH; Raizman NM; Bottino CJ; et al. Unstable distal radial fractures treated with external fixation, a radial column plate, or a volar plate. A prospective randomized trial. J Bone Joint Surg Am. 2009 Jul;91(7):1568-77

Theme 3: Associated Injuries

- Geissler WB, Freeland AE, Savoie FH, McIntyre LW, Whipple TL. Intracarpal soft-tissue lesions associated with an intra-articular fracture of the distal end of the radius. J Bone Joint Surg Am. 1996;78(3):357–365 - PMID 8613442

- Lindau T; Adlercreutz C; Aspenberg P. Peripheral tears of the triangular fibrocartilage complex cause distal radioulnar joint instability after distal radial fractures. J Hand Surg Am. 2000 May;25(3):464-8

- May MM; Lawton JN; Blazar PE. Ulnar styloid fractures associated with distal radius fractures: incidence and implications for distal radioulnar joint instability. J Hand Surg Am. 2002 Nov;27(6):965-71

Theme 4: Outcome Measures

- Macdermid JC; Richards RS; Donner A; et al. Responsiveness of the short form-36, disability of the arm, shoulder, and hand questionnaire, patient-rated wrist evaluation, and physical impairment measurements in evaluating recovery after a distal radius fracture. J Hand Surg Am. 2000 Mar;25(2):330-40 - PMID 10722826

- Mckay SD; Macdermid JC; Roth JH; Richards, RS. Assessment of complications of distal radius fractures and development of a complication checklist. J Hand Surg Am. 2001 Sep;26(5):916-22 - PMID 11561246

Theme 5: Distal radius fractures in the elderly

- Young BT; Rayan GM. Outcome following nonoperative treatment of displaced distal radius fractures in low-demand patients older than 60 years. J Hand Surg Am. 2000 Jan;25(1):19-28 - PMID 10642469

- Jupiter JB; Ring D; Weitzel PP. Surgical treatment of redisplaced fractures of the distal radius in patients older than 60 years. J Hand Surg Am. 2002 Jul;27(4):714-23 - PMID 12132101

- Orbay JL, Fernandez DL. Volar fixed-angle plate fixation for unstable distal radius

fractures in the elderly patient. J Hand Surg Am. 2004 Jan;29(1):96-102 - PMID 14751111

- Diaz-Garcia RJ; Oda T; Shauver MJ; Chung KC. A systematic review of outcomes and complications of treating unstable distal radius fractures in the elderly. J Hand Surg Am. 2011 May;36(5):824-35.e2

of scientific rigor owing to both the era in which they were conceived and methodological limitations inherent in surgical research. Finally, a criticized article may also be highly cited, reflecting dissent with its conclusions rather than praise. For example, Kristiansen and colleagues[8] (#7 most cited, 195 citations) reported accelerated healing of DRFs managed nonoperatively with a bone stimulator compared with a placebo device. This work generated both scientific interest and criticism about conflict of interest and research bias.[9]

The authors identified 5 overarching themes (see **Box 1**): the importance of restoring anatomic alignment, types of hardware to achieve this, injuries associated with DRFs, measuring outcomes after DRFs, and fractures in the elderly.

THEME 1: THE IMPORTANCE OF ANATOMIC ALIGNMENT

Many highly cited articles consider the importance of restoring premorbid anatomy. The earliest treatments encompass some sort of reduction and immobilization.[10,11] Today, the most cited article in DRF research is the classic by Gartland and Werley published in 1951 (#1, 353 citations).[6] This work was important because of its impact on the existing paradigm. DRF was described as "a fracture which continues to be lightly regarded"[6] despite other publications documenting that DRFs were in fact incredibly morbid injuries. Bacorn and Kurtzke (#8, 174 citations) reported on 2000 Workers' Compensation cases of DRFs and found an astounding 97% permanent disability after DRFs, with an average reduction in hand function, or "disability," of 25%.[12] Disability in this article included any loss of volar flexion (95% of cases), but other publications confirmed these findings: Cooney and colleagues[13] (#3, 177 citations) reported on 565 DRFs from 1968 to 1975 and found 177 (31%) had major complications from compression neuropathy, tendon rupture, Volkmann contracture, arthritis, and stiffness. This publication showed that 1 in 3 patients had a major complication in their series. A quote from the article is a call-to-arms: "A total of

31.7% of unsatisfactory results, however, is much too high for a fracture which continues to be *lightly regarded* [italicization added] and for which treatment tends to follow a routine pattern. The fruits of this attitude are apparent when the entire course of the fracture is reviewed."[6]

Gartland and Werley's article gave surgeons a way to combat complications by reporting on which patients will do poorly after DRFs. The investigators followed 80 patients managed nonoperatively for an average of 18 months (>12 months minimum). They measured radial inclination, volar tilt, and radial height in normal and injured wrists and evaluated functional outcomes using a custom tool. They made several contributions by establishing (1) a normal radial inclination of 23° (13°–30°) and volar tilt of 11° (1°–21°), and (2) that deviation from these normal values at fracture union was associated with decreased range of motion, and the worse the deviation, the worse the impairment. They also found that 60% of fractures lost reduction with plaster immobilization and ultimately appeared just as their injury films did. Realizing that plaster immobilization was inadequate led to the subsequent decades of innovation in fixation. Finally, they showed the association between intra-articular fractures and arthritis. They found no arthritis after extra-articular fractures, 11% after nondisplaced intra-articular fractures, and 40% after displaced intra-articular fractures. This work resulted in Knirk and Jupiter's major contribution 3 decades later.[7] Gartland and Werley's results were replicated by subsequent studies (#11, 162 citations).[14]

Surgeons now had an objective goal when treating DRFs. Sarmiento and colleagues[15] (#9, 172 citations) devised specific bracing strategies to maximize anatomic reduction. Cooney and colleagues[16] (#13, 156 citations) reported early external fixation systems to achieve reduction. Lastly, Pogue and colleagues[17] (#23, 101 citations) attempted to understand the biomechanical consequences of not achieving reduction.

If Gartland and Werley paved the way to establishing the new paradigm in DRF treatment, then Knirk and Jupiter indoctrinated it to this day (#2, 342 citations).[7] From a technical standard, the article has several critical methodological flaws when reviewed with 20+ years of hindsight and improvements in imaging.[18] However, it is hard to overstate the impact of this article. It started a decades-long conversation on what factors are important in managing DRFs, and how best to achieve this. Both conversations are still happening today.

The findings of Knirk and Jupiter were replicated by other researchers. Bradway and colleagues[19] (#10, 167 citations) reviewed 16 patients who failed closed reduction and underwent fixation with external fixation, K-wires, or dorsal plates. After an average of 4.8 years of follow-up, patients with a 2-mm step-off at time of union all had arthritis, whereas only 25% had arthritis if the step-off was less than 2 mm. Trumble and colleagues[20] (#12, 156 citations) reported on 43 patients with displaced intra-articular DRFs, with an average of 38 months' follow-up. They found "the degree to which articular step-off, gap between fragments, and radial shortening are improved by surgery is strongly correlated with improved outcome, even when the results are corrected for severity of initial injury."

Knirk and Jupiter established the new standard that precise anatomic reduction is required to prevent arthritis; however, a challenge to this was the recognition that arthritis on radiographs does not always correlate with functional outcomes. Catalano and colleagues[21] (#20, 107 citations) studied 21 patients with at least 1 mm of articular incongruity for an average of 7 years. They found that all patients examined demonstrated good or excellent functional outcome irrespective of radiographic osteoarthritis.[21] The same investigators reevaluated 16 of the original 21 patients 8 years later. Despite the finding of progressive arthritis, there was no correlation between presence or degree of arthritis and function, and all patients maintained a high level of function measured by the Musculoskeletal Functional Assessment score.[22]

The investigators, however, stated that they sought to achieve anatomic alignment to minimize the development of arthritis, even if this arthritis may not be clinically significant.[22] Therefore, 35 years later, the original contribution by Knirk and Jupiter remains important today. Achieving precise articular anatomic alignment to prevent arthritis remains the current standard for treating DRFs. Based on scientific progress, a new standard will likely emerge that adds nuance in precisely how much surgery is needed to achieve how much articular reduction. Indeed, management of DRFs in the elderly is already deviating from management in the young (Theme 5).

THEME 2: TYPES OF HARDWARE

Once the paradigm of restoring precise articular alignment was established, multiple ways of achieving this were tried. Jupiter and colleagues[23] (#26, 96 citations) tried percutaneous biomaterials in a feasibility study. McQueen and colleagues[24] (#27, 96 citations) performed a prospective, randomized trial of how best to manage DRFs that failed closed treatment. Their surgical groups provide an overview of the day's technology, including open reduction, bone grafting, K-wire fixation, and external fixation, with and without mobilization of the wrist for 3 weeks. No plating systems were used. The outcomes correlated only with malunion at the radiocarpal joint, but none of the operative and nonoperative strategies were better than the others at preventing such malunion.

Plating systems represented a technological advance over pins and plaster and external fixation, and dorsal systems were tried first. Two versions have been highly cited: Ring and colleagues[25] (#14, 146 citations) and Carter and colleagues[26] (#17, 133 citations). Concerns over tendon rupture and plate failures were reported by Kambouroglou and Axelrod[27] (#24, 99 citations), urging caution with the new dorsal plates.

Knowing the importance of articular restoration but not having an elegant way to produce it safely was the environment in which Orbay and Fernandez (#4, 256 citations) produced their landmark article introducing volar fixation of DRFs.[28] This innovation was followed by reports of safety and efficacy from independent early adopters. Chung and colleagues[29] (#18, 132 citations) reported on a prospective cohort of patients that showed normalization of patient-reported outcome questionnaires, with infrequent and minor complications. Musgrave and Idler[30] (#30, 86 citations) showed early active range of motion did not harm fracture reduction after volar plate fixation, paving the way for this technology to lead to faster recovery of hand function.

Rozental and colleagues[31] (#24, 99 citations) and Arora and colleagues[32] (#19, 110 citations) also reported their experience with volar plating but had more reserved conclusions. Their articles ushered in several studies comparing volar fixation with other techniques, including several prospective randomized trials. Rozental and colleagues[31] (#21, 106 citations) compared volar plates with pins and plaster using a prospective randomized design and found volar plating provided better functional results in the early postoperative period with fewer complications. Wright and colleagues[33] (#28, 95 citations) compared volar plating with external fixation. They found equivalent final patient-reported outcome scores but better articular congruity, and a faster return to activity and work in the volar plating group. Equivalent long-term functional outcome and earlier functional benefits when comparing the volar plate to external fixation were also shown by Egol and colleagues[34] (#32, 78 citations) and Wei and colleagues[35] (#33, 77 citations).

These early adopters provided safety and efficacy data that assured surgeons to feel comfortable adopting volar plating. The new goal is to strive for precise anatomic reconstruction, and this is most often done with a volar plate. Other modalities, like intrafocal Kapandji pinning in extra-articular fractures in the elderly,[36] or fragment-specific fixation using multiple mini-plates and multiple exposures, have their specific uses given the specific risks of volar plating.

THEME 3: ASSOCIATED INJURIES

Two articles on ulnar-sided injuries after DRFs are seemingly contradictory; however, taken together, they provide nuance to the understanding. Lindau and colleagues (#22, 105 citations) studied 51 young patients with an average age of 41 (range 20–57). Patients were presumed to not have osteoporosis, had isolated displaced DRFs, and were treated by both closed and open procedure. At the time of injury, all patients had wrist arthroscopy to document presence or absence of a triangular fibrocartilage complex (TFCC) tear. Forty-three of 51 patients had some form of tear, and none were treated per protocol. The distal radioulnar joints (DRUJs) were evaluated after a median of 12 months, and clinical outcomes were measured. They found DRUJ instability in 19 patients. Of the 11 patients who had complete TFCC tears at the time of injury, 10 had DRUJ instability (91%). Only 7 of 32 patients (22%) with no tears, or only partial peripheral tears, had DRUJ instability. DRUJ instability was not associated with radiographic findings at the time of fracture or follow-up. Specifically, ulnar styloid fractures were more common in the patients without DRUJ instability. There was no reporting of size or displacement of ulnar styloid fracture. This article replicated the earlier work of Geissler and colleagues[37] (#15, 141 citations) that reported the high frequency of TFCC and other soft tissue injuries in patients with DRFs.

A few years later, May and colleagues[38] (#31, 86 citations) reviewed 166 DRFs in 160 skeletally mature patients with an average age of 41.4 (range 16.8–95.1), including older patients with potentially more brittle bones. They assessed DRUJ instability and the size and degree of displacement of an associated ulnar styloid fracture. They found fractures at the ulnar styloid base or fractures with displacement of more than 2 mm were both risk factors for DRUJ instability after DRFs.

Ulnar-sided injuries to the wrist are common after DRFs. Both peripheral TFCC tears and ulnar styloid fractures, at its base or displaced greater than 2 mm, are associated with DRUJ instability.

Which pathologic condition occurs depends on a variety of factors and may include age-related osteoporosis. When the DRUJ is unstable only in certain positions of forearm rotation, it can be immobilized with casting or radioulnar pinning in the position of stability. When gross instability is present in all positions of forearm rotation, closed management results in persistent instability and therefore needs to be addressed. If there is a large ulnar styloid fracture, it can be reduced and fixated. If instability remains, or there is no ulnar styloid fracture, a peripheral TFCC tear should be suspected and repaired as indicated.[39,40]

THEME 4: MEASURING OUTCOMES

With the great research interest in DRFs came a desire to know which of the patient-reported outcome scales best captures the experience of patients after DRFs. One way of measuring this is the standardized response mean (SRM). This index is one of several effect size indices to gauge the responsiveness of a scale to clinical change experienced and reported by patients. The SRM is calculated by dividing the mean score change by the standard deviation of that change. If 2 patient-reported outcome scales measured the same mean change in hand function after a DRF, the scale with lower variability within a patient cohort would have the higher SRM and be presumably more reliable. Macdermid and colleagues (#6, 203 citations) studied the SRM of the Short Form-36, Disability of the Arm, Shoulder, and Hand (DASH) questionnaire, Patient-Rated Wrist Evaluation (PRWE), and physical impairment measurements in 59 patients treated with both operative and nonoperative techniques. The PRWE was the most responsive (SRM 2.27), followed by the DASH (SRM 2.01). The least responsive was the Short Form-36 (SRM 0.92). The conclusion is that scales more specific to the wrist were more responsive. The patient-reported outcome scales were also highly responsive in the early postoperative period, when physical tests like grip strength could not be performed. The impact of this article, sixth most cited, likely reflects how patient-rated outcomes have become the centerpiece of the outcomes movement, valued by patients and payers alike.[41] Refinement in instruments used to measure patient outcomes will likely be a productive area of future research.[42]

Complication reporting is also unevenly presented in scientific reports. Mckay and colleagues (#34, 74 citations) presented a unique comparison of complications reported by physicians compared with those reported by patients. They found that patients focused on symptoms more than physicians. They proposed a complication checklist that included 3 tiers of severity for each complication.

THEME 5: DISTAL RADIUS FRACTURES IN THE ELDERLY

Recognizing that radiographic outcomes like arthritis and malunion do not correlate with function in young people,[21] surgeons were interested in determining whether articular restoration was necessary for elderly patients. Young and Rayan[43] (#16, 135 citations) studied 25 low-demand patients older than 60 years following nonoperative treatment of DRFs. They confirmed that the radiographic outcome did not correlate with the functional outcome. Eighty-eight percent was able to return to prior activity level or occupation, only 12% having persistent median nerve symptoms, and 4% developing complex regional pain syndrome as reported complications.

Two other articles studied operating on this specific patient population with contradictory results. Jupiter and colleagues[44] (#35, 69 citations) reported fixing 20 patients over the age of 60 years with either dorsal or volar plates. Although reporting good functional outcomes, 6 of 20 plates had to be removed, 1 tendon ruptured, and 1 patient experienced a nonfatal pulmonary embolus. Two years later, Orbay and Fernandez[45] (#5, 218 citations) reported fixing 24 DRFs in 23 patients all over the age of 75 years, using a different technique, the volar fixation system. They reported good maintenance of reduction, no tendon complications, and no plate removals.

In the years following introduction of volar plating in the early 2000s, there was an increase in operative fixation of DRFs nationally.[46]Diaz-Garcia and colleagues[47] (#29, 94 citations) added higher-quality data to this debate with a systematic review of 21 articles. Cast immobilization resulted in fewer complications with no clear clinical inferiority. Ultimately, multicenter clinical trials were necessary to properly answer the question, what is the best way to treat DRFs in elderly patients? Recently, such high-quality multicenter prospective trials were done that suggest patient factors play a larger role than simply patient age in choosing the correct treatment choice.[48,49]

SUMMARY

Tracing the themes through the decades reveals the story of DRF research has loosely followed the *structure of scientific revolutions*,[50] where an existing *paradigm* is challenged when someone identifies an *anomaly* that does not fit within the paradigm. Anomalies are unexpected, and produce a *crisis*, wherein new science is done to work out the anomaly, and ultimately a new paradigm is established. Innovators thrive in crises; they think outside the box, and their solutions are popularized by the early adopters, who prove safety and efficacy for the early and late majority, through the *diffusion of innovation*.[51]

The most cited articles in DRF research represent major contributions when viewed through the lens of the entire field of hand surgery. The authors' review found that high-quality, multi-institution studies by early adopters demonstrating safety and efficacy allowed a *paradigm* shift in the treatment of DRFs.[50,51] Future articles on DRFs will continue to highlight technological breakthroughs by innovators.

REFERENCES

1. To P, Atkinson CT, Lee DH, et al. The most cited articles in hand surgery over the past 20-plus years: a modern-day reading list. J Hand Surg Am 2013;38(5):983–7.
2. Eberlin KR, Labow BI, Upton J, et al. High-impact articles in hand surgery. Hand (N Y) 2012;7(2):157–62.
3. Piolanti N, Poggetti A, Nucci AM, et al. The 50 most cited articles about wrist surgery. Orthop Rev (Pavia) 2018;10:137–40.
4. Phalen GS. The carpal-tunnel syndrome. Seventeen years' experience in diagnosis and treatment of six hundred fifty-four hands. J Bone Joint Surg Am 1966;48(2):211–28.
5. Napier JR. The prehensile movements of the human hand. J Bone Joint Surg Br 1956;38-B(4):902–13.
6. Gartland JJ, Werley CW. Evaluation of healed Colles' fractures. J Bone Joint Surg Am 1951;33-A(4):895–907.
7. Knirk JL, Jupiter JB. Intra-articular fractures of the distal end of the radius in young adults. J Bone Joint Surg Am 1986;68(5):647–59.
8. Kristiansen TK, Ryaby JP, McCabe J, et al. Accelerated healing of distal radial fractures with the use of specific, low-intensity ultrasound. A multicenter, prospective, randomized, double-blind, placebo-controlled study. J Bone Joint Surg Am 1997;79(7):961–73.
9. Starr AJ, Borer DS, Reinert CM, et al. Conflict of interest, bias, and objectivity in research articles. J Bone Joint Surg Am 2001;83-A(9):1429–31.
10. Diaz-Garcia RJ, Chung KC. The evolution of distal radius fracture management: a historical treatise. Hand Clin 2012;28(2):105–11.
11. Colles A. On the fracture of the carpal extremity of the radius. Edinb Med. Surg. J. 1814;10:182–6.
12. Bacorn RW, Kurtzke JF. Colles' fracture; a study of two thousand cases from the New York State Workmen's Compensation Board. J Bone Joint Surg Am 1953;35-A:643–58.
13. Cooney WP 3rd, Dobyns JH, Linscheid RL. Complications of Colles' fractures. J Bone Joint Surg Am 1980;62(4):613–9.
14. Mcqueen M, Caspers J. Colles fracture: does the anatomical result affect the final function? J Bone Joint Surg Br 1988;70(4):649–51.
15. Sarmiento A, Pratt GW, Berry NC, et al. Colles' fractures. Functional bracing in supination. J Bone Joint Surg Am 1975;57(3):311–7.
16. Cooney WP 3rd, Linscheid RL, Dobyns JH. External pin fixation for unstable Colles' fractures. J Bone Joint Surg Am 1979;61(6A):840–5.
17. Pogue DJ, Viegas SF, Patterson RM, et al. Effects of distal radius fracture malunion on wrist joint mechanics. J Hand Surg Am 1990;15(5):721–7.
18. Haus BM, Jupiter JB. Intra-articular fractures of the distal end of the radius in young adults: reexamined as evidence-based and outcomes medicine. J Bone Joint Surg Am 2009;91(12):2984–91.
19. Bradway JK, Amadio PC, Cooney WP. Open reduction and internal fixation of displaced, comminuted intra-articular fractures of the distal end of the radius. J Bone Joint Surg Am 1989;71(6):839–47.
20. Trumble TE, Schmitt SR, Vedder NB. Factors affecting functional outcome of displaced intra-articular distal radius fractures. J Hand Surg Am 1994;19(2):325–40.
21. Catalano LW, Cole RJ, Gelberman RH, et al. Displaced intra-articular fractures of the distal aspect of the radius. Long-term results in young adults after open reduction and internal fixation. J Bone Joint Surg Am 1997;79(9):1290–302.
22. Goldfarb CA, Rudzki JR, Catalano LW, et al. Fifteen-year outcome of displaced intra-articular fractures of the distal radius. J Hand Surg Am 2006;31(4):633–9.
23. Jupiter JB, Winters S, Sigman S, et al. Repair of five distal radius fractures with an investigational cancellous bone cement: a preliminary report. J Orthop Trauma 1997;11(2):110–6.
24. McQueen MM, Hajducka C, Court-Brown CM. Redisplaced unstable fractures of the distal radius: a prospective randomised comparison of four methods of treatment. J Bone Joint Surg Br 1996;78(3):404–9.
25. Ring D, Jupiter JB, Brennwald J, et al. Prospective multicenter trial of a plate for dorsal fixation of distal radius fractures. J Hand Surg Am 1997;22(5):777–84.
26. Carter PR, Frederick HA, Laseter GF. Open reduction and internal fixation of unstable distal radius fractures with a low-profile plate: a multicenter study of 73 fractures. J Hand Surg Am 1998;23(2):300–7.

27. Kambouroglou GK, Axelrod TS. Complications of the AO/ASIF titanium distal radius plate system (pi plate) in internal fixation of the distal radius: a brief report. J Hand Surg Am 1998;23(4):737–41.

28. Orbay JL, Fernandez DL. Volar fixation for dorsally displaced fractures of the distal radius: a preliminary report. J Hand Surg Am 2002;27(2):205–15.

29. Chung KC, Watt AJ, Kotsis SV, et al. Treatment of unstable distal radial fractures with the volar locking plating system. J Bone Joint Surg Am 2006;88(12): 2687–94.

30. Musgrave DS, Idler RS. Volar fixation of dorsally displaced distal radius fractures using the 2.4-mm locking compression plates. J Hand Surg Am 2005;30(4):743–9.

31. Rozental TD, Blazar PE, Franko OI, et al. Functional outcomes for unstable distal radial fractures treated with open reduction and internal fixation or closed reduction and percutaneous fixation. J Bone Joint Surg Am 2009;91(8):1837–46.

32. Arora R, Lutz M, Hennerbichler A, et al. Complications following internal fixation of unstable distal radius fracture with a palmar locking-plate. J Orthop Trauma 2007;21(5):316–22.

33. Wright TW, Horodyski M, Smith DW. Functional outcome of unstable distal radius fractures: ORIF with a volar fixed-angle tine plate versus external fixation. J Hand Surg Am 2005;30(2):289–99.

34. Egol K, Walsh M, Tejwani N, et al. Bridging external fixation and supplementary Kirschner-wire fixation versus volar locked plating for unstable fractures of the distal radius: a randomised, prospective trial. J Bone Joint Surg Br 2008;90(9):1214–21.

35. Wei DH, Raizman NM, Bottino CJ, et al. Unstable distal radial fractures treated with external fixation, a radial column plate, or a volar plate. J Bone Joint Surg Am 2009;91(7):1568–77.

36. Greatting MD, Bishop AT. Intrafocal (Kapandji) pinning of unstable fractures of the distal radius. Orthop Clin North Am 1993;24(2):301–7.

37. Geissler WB, Freeland AE, Savoie FH, et al. Intracarpal soft-tissue lesions associated with an intraarticular fracture of the distal end of the radius. J Bone Joint Surg Am 1996;78(3):357–65.

38. May MM, Lawton JN, Blazar PE. Ulnar styloid fractures associated with distal radius fractures: incidence and implications for distal radioulnar joint instability. J Hand Surg Am 2002;27(6):965–71.

39. Sammer DM, Shah HM, Shauver MJ, et al. The effect of ulnar styloid fractures on patient-rated outcomes after volar locking plating of distal radius fractures. J Hand Surg Am 2009;34(9):1595–602.

40. Sammer DM, Chung KC. Management of the distal radioulnar joint and ulnar styloid fracture. Hand Clin 2012;28(2):199–206.

41. Shauver MJ, Chung KC. The Michigan Hand Outcomes Questionnaire after 15 years of field trial. Plast Reconstr Surg 2013;131(5):779e.

42. Sandvall B, Okoroafor UC, Gerull W, et al. Minimal clinically important difference for PROMIS physical function in patients with distal radius fractures. J Hand Surg Am 2019;44(6):454.e1.

43. Young BT, Rayan GM. Outcome following nonoperative treatment of displaced distal radius fractures in low-demand patients older than 60 years. J Hand Surg Am 2000;25(1):19–28.

44. Jupiter JB, Ring D, Weitzel PP. Surgical treatment of redisplaced fractures of the distal radius in patients older than 60 years. J Hand Surg Am 2002;27(4): 714–23.

45. Orbay JL, Fernandez DL. Volar fixed-angle plate fixation for unstable distal radius fractures in the elderly patient. J Hand Surg Am 2004;29(1): 96–102.

46. Chung KC, Shauver MJ, Birkmeyer JD. Trends in the United States in the treatment of distal radial fractures in the elderly. J Bone Joint Surg Am 2009; 91(8):1868–73.

47. Diaz-Garcia RJ, Oda T, Shauver MJ, et al. A systematic review of outcomes and complications of treating unstable distal radius fractures in the elderly. J Hand Surg Am 2011;36(5):824.e2.

48. Hooper RC, Zhou N, Wang L, et al. Pre-injury activity predicts outcomes following distal radius fractures in patients age 60 and older. PLoS One 2020; 15(5):e0232684.

49. Chung KC, Cho HE, Kim Y, et al. Assessment of anatomic restoration of distal radius fractures among older adults: a secondary analysis of a randomized clinical trial. JAMA Netw Open 2020;3(1): e1919433.

50. Kuhn, T. S. The structure of scientific revolutions. (1962).

51. Rogers, E. M. Diffusion of Innovation. (1962).

Nuances of Radiographic Assessment of Distal Radius Fractures to Avoid Missed Fragments

Jeremy E. Raducha, MD[a],*, Christopher J. Got, MD[b]

KEYWORDS

- Distal radius • Radiographs • Computed tomography

KEY POINTS

- Most fracture fragments and characteristics can be assessed on plain radiographs using various radiographic views and measurements.
- Particular attention should be paid to the volar ulnar rim fragment.
- The dorsal ulnar corner and intra-articular free fragment typically require computed tomographic scan for accurate evaluation.
- Several fluoroscopic views are described to evaluate intra-articular and dorsal cortex screw penetration, which should be used to help prevent complications and revision surgery.

INTRODUCTION

In the not so distant past, the radiographic evaluation of fractures, including wrist/distal radius fractures, was limited to fairly low-quality, hard images that were more difficult to interpret. We now have extremely high-tech imaging capabilities that are beginning to even allow live motion tracking modes with true 3-dimensional (3D) reconstructions. However, even though this technology allows us to better visualize these fracture patterns, understanding exactly what you are seeing can be much more difficult. There also remains considerable debate about which fractures require surgical fixation and what are the true long-term consequences of malreduction. The classic study by Knirk and Jupiter[1] found a 94% correlation between greater than 1-mm articular step-off on plain radiographs at the time of injury and radiographic signs of degenerative disease at long-term follow-up, with 86% being symptomatic if the initial step-off was greater than 2 mm. Numerous other articles have established different cutoffs for acceptable amounts of radial shortening, dorsal/volar tilt, coronal shift, and so forth. Now studies using advanced imaging and patient-reported outcomes are revisiting these cutoffs to determine if there is a link between the accuracy of reduction and functional outcomes.[2–4]

It is generally thought that radial shortening greater than 5 mm, ulnar variance greater than 3 mm, dorsal tilt greater than 10°, or intra-articular step-off greater than 2 mm are indications for operative intervention in younger, active adults.[5] Debating the true operative indications in various groups of patients is beyond the scope of this article, but with such small variations from normal being acceptable, it can be difficult to determine the appropriateness of the reduction. The authors focus on the various imaging studies

[a] Department of Orthopedics, Brown University, Lifespan Inc, Rhode Island Hospital, Miriam Hospital, 593 Eddy Street, Providence, RI 02905, USA; [b] Department of Orthopedics, Brown University, University Orthopedics Inc, Lifespan Rhode Island Hospital, Miriam Hospital, 593 Eddy Street, Providence, RI 02905, USA
* Corresponding author.
E-mail address: Jeremy.raducha@gmail.com

Hand Clin 37 (2021) 197–204
https://doi.org/10.1016/j.hcl.2021.02.002
0749-0712/21/© 2021 Elsevier Inc. All rights reserved.

and views that can be used preoperatively, intraoperatively, and postoperatively to determine if the reduction is acceptable and evaluate the safety of the plate/screw position. However, to best understand what is being seen in each image, distal radius anatomy and common fracture patterns encountered must first be discussed.

Anatomy

The distal end of the radius forms the main proximal component for the radiocarpal joint through its biconcave articulation with the scaphoid and lunate. It supports ~80% of the load through an ulnar neutral wrist.[6] The radial aspect of the bone extends more distally at the styloid, giving the wrist joint a distal-radial to proximal-ulnar orientation, and accounting for the radial height and inclination. The articular surface also tilts volarly in the sagittal plane, accounting for the radial tilt (**Fig. 1**). The "normal" radial height is ~11 mm (8–18 mm) with ~22° (13°–30°) of inclination and ~11° (0°–28°) volar tilt, although there is a wide range of "normal" measurements (**Fig. 2**). Because of the volar tilt, the volar rim will sit proximal to the dorsal rim and can create overlap on posteroanterior (PA) imaging, making it difficult to interpret. Ulnarly, the sigmoid notch articulates with the ulnar head, forming the distal radioulnar joint (DRUJ). This joint can have multiple normal variations in the coronal and axial planes (**Fig. 3**), which can make it difficult to determine what is "normal" in each particular patient.[7,8] These variations highlight the usefulness of obtaining contralateral films to evaluate a patient's uninjured anatomy and, as is the case with the DRUJ, prevent malreduction.

There are strong volar ligaments attaching the radius and ulna to the carpal bones, namely, the long and short radiolunate, and radioscaphocapitate ligaments. Deep and superficial radioulnar ligaments as well as others in conjunction with the fibrocartilaginous disc make up the triangular fibrocartilage complex (TFCC). The interosseous membrane, mainly the distal oblique band, adds to the additional stability of the DRUJ. All of these ligaments can affect fracture pattern, and their integrity should be considered during fracture management.

The "Watershed Line" is a theoretic line that represents the most volar aspect of the distal radius and is an important landmark for surgical intervention, as it has been shown that plates positioned more distal to this point have an increased rate of flexor tendon irritation and injury.[9] It can be identified on a true lateral radiograph of the wrist, or clinically, it can be found just distal to the pronator quadratus at the level of the ulnar prominence.[10]

Typical Fracture Patterns

There are several classification schemes, including the eponym, Mayo, Melone, AO, Fernandez, Frykman, and Fragment specific classifications; all attempt to group common fracture patterns or pieces to ease understanding. Most have shown poor interobserver reliability and poor correlation between fracture pattern and postinjury functional outcomes.[11–13] However, one can use these classifications to better recognize common fracture patterns. When considering intra-articular fractures, there are 5 main fragments of the distal radius: styloid, volar ulnar rim, dorsal ulnar corner, dorsal wall, and a central, free articular fragment.[14] Most intra-articular fracture lines concentrate around Listers tubercle. These fractures often propagate along the interval between the radioscaphoid and

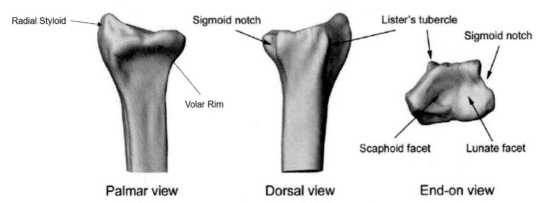

Fig. 1. Representation of the relevant components distal radius anatomy. (Reproduced with permission from: Madant R. The Use of Radiostereometric Analysis in Fractures of the Distal Radius: From Phantom Models to Clinical Application. https://www.utupub.fi/handle/10024/66700).

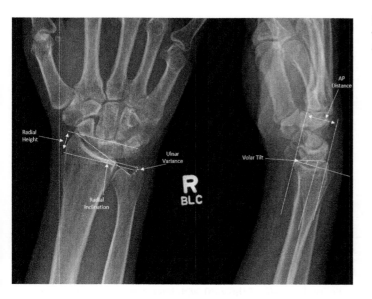

Fig. 2. Radiographic PA and lateral views of the wrist with common alignment measurements.

radiolunate facets and can be associated with significant comminution of the dorsal wall.[13]

Plain Radiographs

The wrist series of plain radiographs typically includes 3 views: PA, lateral, and oblique (**Fig. 4**). As with all radiographs, the reviewer must extrapolate the lines and shadowing on this 2-dimensional image to discern how this correlates with the 3D object it portrays. Radiographs performed in the setting of a widely displaced fracture are often more difficult to interpret. However, when referenced with post reduction imaging, these radiographs may prove useful to appreciate additional fragments as well as the orientation of

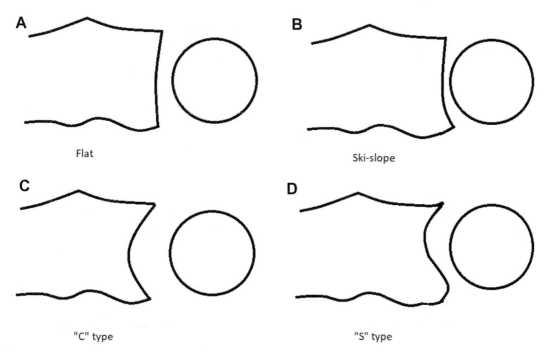

Fig. 3. Variations of DRUJ anatomy. (*A*) A flat sigmoid notch, (*B*) a ski-slope sigmoid notch, (*C*) a "C" type sigmoid notch, (*D*) an "S"-type sigmoid notch. (*Data from* Tolat AR, Stanley JK, Trail IA. A cadaveric study of the anatomy and stability of the distal radioulnar joint in the coronal and transverse planes. *J Hand Surg Eur Vol.* 1996;21(5):587-594. https://doi.org/10.1016/S0266-7681(96)80136-7.)

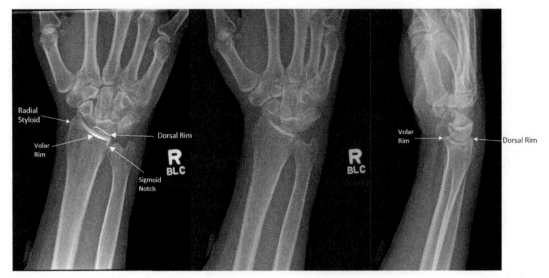

Fig. 4. Standard PA, oblique, and lateral radiographic views of the wrist with important structures labeled.

proposed hardware. Once reduced, the first step is to establish the quality of radiographs being evaluated. The PA radiograph should be taken with the shoulder at 90° abduction and elbow at 90° of flexion with a neutral forearm and the projection centered on the capitate. The lateral radiograph should be taken with the shoulder adducted, elbow at 90° flexion, and hand in the same plane as the humerus. These positions are important, as rotation of the forearm by just 5° has been shown to change the measured volar tilt by 1.6°, which is increased with supination and decreased with pronation.[11] With appropriate radiographs, an enormous amount of information is discernible without advanced imaging.

The PA radiograph is best at viewing the radial styloid fragment. It is also used to measure the radial height, ulnar variance, radial inclination, and DRUJ articulation. The radial height is the measured distance between a line drawn tangential to the radial styloid tip and one drawn tangential to the distal edge of the ulnar head (**Fig. 2**).[11] Radial shortening has been shown in a cadaver study to have the greatest distortion of the TFCC and effect on DRUJ kinematics by tightening the DRUJ ligaments and reducing supination/pronation.[15] Ulnar variance, sometimes confused with radial height, is also measured on a PA radiograph. It is the distance between the line tangential to the lunate facet of the radius and the one tangential to the distal aspect of the ulnar head. Ulnar positive variance can also be associated with alteration of DRUJ kinematics as well as ulnar abutment of the carpus, which can lead to pain and decreased grip strength. Radial inclination is the angle between the line drawn from the tip of the styloid to the medial articular corner and a line drawn perpendicular to the axis of the radius.[11] Pogue and colleagues[16] found that radial inclination decreased below 0° when radial shortening exceeded 4 mm. Radial and ulnar translation of the distal fracture fragments is also best evaluated on the PA radiograph.

The lateral radiograph is best to visualize the dorsal wall and volar rim fragments. Dorsal subluxation of the ulnar head also suggests displacement of a dorsal ulnar corner fragment or DRUJ instability. It is also used to make several measurements. The volar tilt is the angle between the line drawn between the distal volar and dorsal rims and a line perpendicular to the radial shaft. The radial shaft, lunate, capitate, and third metacarpal should all align on the lateral view, and the carpal alignment can be measured as the angle between the long axes of the radius and the capitate. If those axes do not intersect within the level of the carpus, the radius is malaligned, and the distal carpal row is compensates for the change in tilt.[11] It has also been shown that dorsal tilt greater than 15° was not possible without an ulnar styloid fracture or injury to the TFCC,[16] so it is important to be vigilant for a TFCC injury and/or DRUJ instability in patients with significant initial dorsal angulation of their fractures. The anterior-posterior (AP) distance and teardrop angle can also be measured on the lateral radiograph. The AP distance is simply the distance between the apex of the volar and dorsal lips of the lunate facet, measured with 10° of lateral tilt. An increase in this distance indicates discontinuity of the dorsal and volar rim and can be the only evidence of sigmoid notch displacement.[17] The teardrop is a U-shaped structure on the 10° tilt lateral view, which represents the volar lip of the lunate facet. The teardrop angle is measured between the axis of the radial shaft and a line drawn through the central axis of the teardrop, normally ~70°.[4,14,17] With articular impaction and dissociation of the volar and dorsal radial cortices, this volar lip fragment can rotate dorsally into the comminuted metaphysis. A decrease in this angle indicates residual displacement of the volar rim fragment and articular surface, which may not be recognized initially if other alignment parameters are acceptable.[4]

The standard oblique radiograph is taken with the arm positioned similarly to the lateral, except the forearm and hand are pronated 45°. This position provides an improved view of the dorsal ulnar corner fragment. The central articular fragment is not well visualized on any radiographic views, making it difficult to assess its reduction without the use of advanced imaging.

Fluoroscopy

Intraoperatively, it can be difficult to evaluate fracture reduction and plate/screw position clinically. Assessing the articular surface clinically requires a second dorsal incision and arthrotomy or wrist arthroscopy, as the stout volar radiocarpal ligaments should not be violated. To properly assess these variables, fluoroscopy has become a mainstay of the operating room, and more recently, rotational/3D fluoroscopic use has also been described.

The standard PA, oblique, and lateral fluoroscopic views are useful to assess radial height, inclination, ulnar variance, and volar tilt, but do not allow accurate evaluation of articular step-off, or screw penetration of the joint or dorsal radial cortex. Because of the volar tilt of the articular surface, PA views show radiographic overlap of the volar rim on the dorsal cortex. By angling the fluoroscopic beam to match the volar tilt of the radius, there is a greater ability to assess the true joint line and articular step-off.[18] When assessing screw penetration of the articular surface, the 20° elevated lateral view can be useful, as it positions the x-ray beam to shoot tangentially to the scaphoid facet surface (**Fig. 5**).

Penetration of screws through the dorsal cortex of the radius increases the risk of extensor tendon irritation, and measuring screw length with a depth gauge can be difficult with dorsal comminution. Stoops and colleagues[19] showed as many as 9.1% of volar locking plate screws were on average 2 mm long if using the length measured with the depth gauge. Checking the screw lengths with standard fluoroscopic views can also be

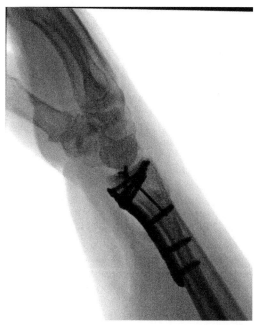

Fig. 5. 20° tilt lateral view, demonstrated on an intraoperative fluoroscopic image to assess screw penetration of the articular surface.

difficult because Lister tubercle protrudes dorsally to obscure the lateral view. To overcome these difficulties, 2 particular fluoroscopic views have been described. The dorsal tangential view, or skyline view, is performed with the elbow flexed 70° to 75°, forearm fully supinated, and wrist fully flexed[19] (**Fig. 6**). This position allows an axial view of the distal radius to assess dorsal screw penetration and has been found to detect ~25%

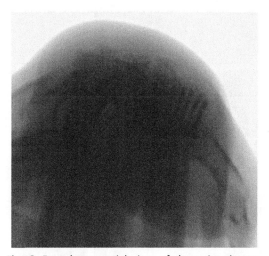

Fig. 6. Dorsal tangential view of the wrist, demonstrated on an intraoperative fluoroscopic image to assess screw penetration of the dorsal cortex.

more prominent screw than standard fluoroscopic views.[20] Other studies have shown it to be highly sensitive, with a 91% negative predictive value and 91% accuracy.[21,22] The carpal shoot-through view is another option to assess dorsal screw penetration, although not as thoroughly studied as the dorsal tangential view. The arm is positioned the same as the dorsal tangential view, but the wrist is extended instead of flexed in order to overcome the difficulty of hyperflexion in patients with a large soft tissue envelope or swelling. It has been found to require fewer images to obtain a correct view compared with the dorsal tangential view with a sensitivity of 86% and specificity of 84% compared with 75% and 85%, respectively, for the dorsal tangential view ($P<.001$ and $P<.001$).[19]

Intraoperatively, 360° or 3D fluoroscopy has also been used in an attempt to more accurately assess fracture reduction and screw position. It has been found to have similar negative predictive value, 93%, and accuracy, 93%, and similarly reduce the risk of dorsal screw penetration compared with the dorsal tangential view.[21] However, it requires a more skilled technician to perform, along with higher cost and radiation exposure. In a recent meta-analysis of 27 studies evaluating multiple forms of imaging to assess dorsal and articular screw penetration, oblique pronated and AP views had the lowest interobserver reliability, whereas the dorsal tangential view had the highest sensitivity for assessing dorsal penetration. CT scans were found to most accurately assess articular screw penetration and are actually used as the standard many of these other imaging modalities are compared with for assessing reduction and screw penetration.[22]

Computed Tomography

Computed tomography (CT) can be a useful tool to assess fracture fragments and reduction preoperatively, intraoperatively, and postoperatively. Preoperatively, there are 2 main fragments that the CT scan helps most with assessing, the dorsal ulnar corner and the central articular fragment (**Fig. 7**). The dorsal ulnar corner can involve 10% to 36% of the lunate facet articular surface (3.8–13.6 mm in AP width) and up to 50% of the sigmoid notch articular surface.[23,24] The dorsal ulnar corner can be a fairly large piece whose

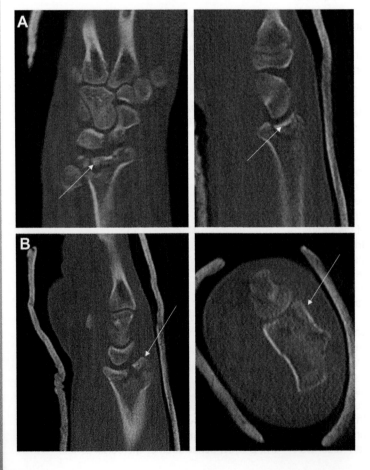

Fig. 7. CT scan of the wrist highlighting the benefit of this imaging study when assessing the intra-articular free fragment [*arrows*] (*A*) and dorsal ulnar corner [*arrows*] (*B*).

displacement or malreduction could affect the DRUJ or radiocarpal joint. It has been shown that failure to capture this piece with at least 1 screw from a volar locking plate resulted in postoperative displacement seen on imaging.[23] However, there has been some debate in the literature as to whether the reduction of this piece truly affects final outcomes.[23,25,26]

Radiographs have also been shown to underestimate the level of comminution and degrees of articular step-off, including the central fragment and lunate fossa compared with CT scans.[27,28] For this reason, some have proposed even using CT scans intraoperatively to assess fracture reduction and screw penetration, much like is done with spinal instrumentation. Halvachizadeh and colleagues[29] compared intraoperative CT scans to conventional fluoroscopy during distal radius fixation. They found the CT scans were used more commonly in AO Type C fractures, had a similar operative time, and allowed 25% of screws to be resized after intraoperative scan. However, the rate of revision surgery was similar to the fluoroscopic group, and the radiation exposure was higher, leading them to conclude it may not be worth the risks and costs.

Postoperatively, CT scans can be used to assess reduction or evaluate healing, and now the advent of 3D CT scans allows the calculation of joint space and surface area to assess degenerative changes. One such evaluation showed loss of 3D joints space at the lunate facet at an average of 8 years postdistal radius fracture with relative preservation of the radioscaphoid facet and DRUJ, which may lead to altered joint mechanics and posttraumatic arthritis.[3]

Alternatives

The cost and radiation exposure to CT scan have led some investigators to investigate imaging alternatives. Digital tomosynthesis or trispiral tomography acquires a series of images over a limited angular range, allowing a 3D image with a lower number of slices. It has been shown to be less than 50% of the cost and less than 50% of the radiation compared with conventional CT but has similar ability to assess articular step-off.[30,31]

Ultrasound has also been used to assess dorsal screw penetration intraoperatively and had been found to be similarly accurate to dorsal tangential views when assess the second and third dorsal compartments, and even superior when assessing the fourth dorsal compartment.[32] It is low cost and does not use radiation; however, as with the use of ultrasound in all other applications, it is highly operator dependent.

SUMMARY

Overall, because of its anatomy, imaging of the distal radius provides some unique challenges to accurately evaluate fracture fragments and reductions. With the use of standard and additional radiographic/fluoroscopic views, most fracture characteristics can be determined if inspected carefully. The addition of 2dimensional and 3D CT scans can help better evaluate difficult-to-assess central joint depression and dorsal ulnar fragments. Using these tools in combination with surgeon experience can ensure appropriate nonsurgical and surgical management.

CLINICS CARE POINTS

- Most fracture fragments and characteristics can be assessed on plain radiographs using various radiographic views and measurements.
- Particular attention should be paid to the volar ulnar rim fragment.
- The dorsal ulnar corner and intra-articular free fragment typically require CT scan for accurate evaluation
- Several fluoroscopic views are described to evaluate intra-articular and dorsal cortex screw penetration, which should be used to help prevent complications and revision surgery.

DISCLOSURE

The authors have nothing to disclose.

REFERENCES

1. Knirk JL, Jupiter JB. Intra-articular fractures of the distal end of the radius in young adults. J Bone Joint Surg Am 1986;68(5):647.

2. Wollstein R, Allon R, Zvi Y, et al. Association between functional outcomes and radiographic reduction following surgery for distal radius fractures. J Hand Surg Asian Pac Vol 2019;24(3):258–63.

3. Lalone EA, MacDermid J, King G, et al. The effect of distal radius fractures on 3-dimensional joint congruency. J Hand Surg Am 2020. https://doi.org/10.1016/j.jhsa.2020.05.027.

4. Haus BM, Jupiter JB. Intra-articular fractures of the distal end of the radius in young adults: reexamined as evidence-based and outcomes medicine. J Bone Joint Surg Am 2009;91(12):2984–91.

5. Bartolotta RJ, Daniels SP, Verret CI, et al. Current fixation options for elbow, forearm, wrist, and hand fractures. Semin Musculoskelet Radiol 2019;23(2):109–25.

6. Palmer AK, Werner FW. The triangular fibrocartilage complex of the wrist—anatomy and function. J Hand Surg Am 1981;6(2):153–62.

7. Tolat AR, Stanley JK, Trail IA. A cadaveric study of the anatomy and stability of the distal radioulnar joint in the coronal and transverse planes. J Hand Surg Eur Vol 1996;21(5):587–94.

8. Huang JI, Hanel DP. Anatomy and biomechanics of the distal radioulnar joint. Hand Clin 2012;28(2):157–63.

9. Soong M, Earp BE, Bishop G, et al. Volar locking plate implant prominence and flexor tendon rupture. J Bone Joint Surg Am 2011;93(4):328–35.

10. Bergsma M, Doornberg JN, Borghorst A, et al. The watershed line of the distal radius: cadaveric and imaging study of anatomical landmarks. J Wrist Surg 2020;09(01):044–51.

11. Ng CY, McQueen MM. What are the radiological predictors of functional outcome following fractures of the distal radius? J Bone Joint Surg Br 2011;93B(2):145–50.

12. Sipakarn Y, Niempoog S, Boontanapibul K. The comparative study of reliability and reproducibility of distal radius' fracture classification among: AO frykman and Fernandez classification systems. J Med Assoc Thail 2013;96(1):52–7. Available at: https://pubmed.ncbi.nlm.nih.gov/23720978/. Accessed September 28, 2020.

13. Li S, Zhang YQ, Wang GH, et al. Melone's concept revisited in comminuted distal radius fractures: the three-dimensional CT mapping. J Orthop Surg Res 2020;15(1). https://doi.org/10.1186/s13018-020-01739-x.

14. Rhee PC, Medoff RJ, Shin AY. Complex distal radius fractures: an anatomic algorithm for surgical management. J Am Acad Orthop Surg 2017;25(2):77–88.

15. Adams BD. Effects of radial deformity on distal radioulnar joint mechanics. J Hand Surg Am 1993;18(3):492–8.

16. Pogue DJ, Viegas SF, Patterson RM, et al. Effects of distal radius fracture malunion on wrist joint mechanics. J Hand Surg Am 1990;15(5):721–7.

17. Medoff RJ. Essential radiographic evaluation for distal radius fractures. Hand Clin 2005;21(3):279–88.

18. Beldner S, Rabinovich RV, Polatsch DB. Intraoperative tilted posteroanterior view for the measurement of distal radius articular step-off. J Wrist Surg 2019;08(04):300–4.

19. Stoops TK, Santoni BG, Clark NM, et al. Sensitivity and specificity of skyline and carpal shoot-through fluoroscopic views of volar plate fixation of the distal radius: a cadaveric investigation of dorsal cortex screw penetration. Hand 2017;12(6):551–6.

20. Ozer K, Toker S. Dorsal tangential view of the wrist to detect screw penetration to the dorsal cortex of the distal radius after volar fixed-angle plating. Hand 2011;6(2):190–3.

21. Langerhuizen DWG, Bergsma M, Selles CA, et al. Diagnosis of dorsal screw penetration after volar plating of a distal radial fracture. Bone Joint J 2020;102-B(7):874–80.

22. Maschke SD, Evans PJ, Schub D, et al. Radiographic evaluation of dorsal screw penetration after volar fixed-angle plating of the distal radius: a cadaveric study. Hand 2007;2(3):144–50.

23. Miyashima Y, Kaneshiro Y, Yano K, et al. Size and stabilization of the dorsoulnar fragment in AO C3-type distal radius fractures. Injury 2019;50(11):2004–8.

24. Zimmer J, Atwood DN, Lovy AJ, et al. Characterization of the dorsal ulnar corner in distal radius fractures in postmenopausal females: implications for surgical decision making. J Hand Surg Am 2020;45(6):495–502.

25. Kim JK, Cho SW. The effects of a displaced dorsal rim fracture on outcomes after volar plate fixation of a distal radius fracture. Injury 2012;43(2):143–6.

26. Dy C, Wolfe S, Jupiter J, et al. Distal radius fractures: strategic alternatives to volar plate fixation. Instr Course Lect 2014;63:27–37.

27. Pruitt DL, Gilula LA, Manske PR, et al. Computed tomography scanning with image reconstruction in evaluation of distal radius fractures. J Hand Surg Am 1994;19(5):720–7.

28. Cole RJ, Bindra RR, Evanoff BA, et al. Radiographic evaluation of osseous displacement following intra-articular fractures of the distal radius: reliability of plain radiography versus computed tomography. J Hand Surg Am 1997;22(5):792–800.

29. Halvachizadeh S, Berk T, Pieringer A, et al. Is the additional effort for an intraoperative CT scan justified for distal radius fracture fixations? A comparative clinical feasibility study. J Clin Med 2020;9(7):2254.

30. Freedman DM, Dawdle J, Glickel SZ, et al. Tomography versus computed tomography for assessing step off in intraarticular distal radial fractures. Clin Orthop Relat Res 1999;361:199–204.

31. Hashimoto S, Yamazaki H, Hayashi M, et al. Radiographic change in articular reduction after volar locking plating for intra-articular distal radius fractures. J Hand Surg Am 2020;45(4):335–40.

32. Gurbuz Y, Kucuk L, Gunay H, et al. Comparison of ultrasound and dorsal horizon radiographic view for the detection of dorsal screw penetration. Acta Orthop Traumatol Turc 2017;51(6):448–50.

How to Treat Distal Radius Fractures

Right Patient, Right Care, Right Time, and Right Cost

Paul M. Inclan, MD, Christopher J. Dy, MD, MPH*

KEYWORDS

- Distal radius fracture • Volar plate fixation • Cost-effective care

KEY POINTS

- Operative management of distal radius fractures is determined by radiographic (volar tilt, radial height, articular congruity, carpal alignment) and patient (activity level, age, preference) factors.
- Although many options exist for operative fixation, volar plates represent the mainstay of operative management.
- Cost-effective care requires judicious use of postoperative rehabilitation and consideration of implant and facility cost while delivering care.

INTRODUCTION

Distal radius fractures are the most common upper extremity fracture, affecting young patients experiencing high-velocity trauma and older adults subjected to lower-energy injuries.[1,2] Therefore, treatment of a distal radius fracture, intended to optimize the patient's short- and long-term outcomes, requires understanding of the fracture, any associated injuries, and the patient that has suffered the injury.

The goal of distal radius fracture management is to provide a treatment that optimizes function in an acceptable timeframe while minimizing the risks of complications. One of the main challenges faced by surgeons is predicting which fractures will heal in a position that yields reasonable function. Although it is apparent from the literature that malunion of the distal radius is better tolerated than malunion in other bones,[3,4] there is a threshold of malalignment that may have negative implications on function, particularly in younger patients. Residual articular incongruity correlates with the individual's subsequent risk of post-traumatic osteoarthritis yet does not seem to correlate with functional outcomes following management.[5,6] As such, radiographic outcomes must be tempered with functional and patient-reported measures.[7]

Finally, a systems-based approach to distal radius fractures also requires considerations of the costs associated with perioperative care and postoperative therapy. Nonoperative management, with lower initial cost than operative fixation, must be considered in the context of prolonged functional recovery and the potential, albeit unlikely, need for malunion correction.[8] If surgery is selected, there is significant variability in cost and use of internal fixation, closed reduction and percutaneous pinning, and external fixation.[9]

RIGHT PATIENT

The most influential patient-specific characteristic to consider in the treatment of distal radius fractures is patient age. Advanced age represents the greatest risk factor for secondary displacement following closed reduction of a distal radius

Department of Orthopaedic Surgery, Washington University in St. Louis, 660 Euclid Avenue, Campus Box 8233, St Louis, MO 63110, USA
* Corresponding author.
E-mail address: dyc@wustl.edu

Hand Clin 37 (2021) 205–214
https://doi.org/10.1016/j.hcl.2021.02.003
0749-0712/21/© 2021 Elsevier Inc. All rights reserved.

fracture,[10] with the risk for secondary displacement in geriatric populations approaching 90%.[11] As such, elderly patients require close clinical follow-up and serial radiographs to ensure maintenance of reduction.[12] However, numerous studies in older adults indicate that satisfactory functional outcomes is obtained with nonoperative management,[8] regardless of the presence of radiographic malunion,[12] complicating the decision to pursue operative intervention in this patient population. Moreover, chronologic age may differ significantly from physiologic age; therefore, patient-specific function and functional demands should be considered. Although many surgeons are likely to use baseline activity level as a decision-making factor, regardless of age, it should be noted that malunions are well-tolerated even in high activity older adults.[13] Given such equipoise, American Academy of Orthopedic Surgeons (AAOS) clinical practice guidelines could not recommend for or against operative management of distal radius fractures in patients older than the age of 55.[14]

In younger (<55 years) patients, meta-analysis indicate grip strength and DASH scores may be superior in fractures treated with internal fixation,[15] slightly changing the calculus for operative intervention. Practically, surgeons are more likely to guide younger patients for operative management.[16] Given the superior short-term functional outcomes with operative fixation,[8] surgery may be considered to allow for earlier return-to-work[17] and return-to-sport.[18] Surgical treatment of distal radius fractures may also be particularly advantageous in the multiply injured patient.[19] Earlier weight-bearing is important, given the likely need for crutches or other assistive devices in the setting of concurrent lower extremity injuries. For this reason, concurrent long bone injuries or significant intra-abdominal and chest wall injuries complicating mobilization are considered a relative indication for operative fixation of a distal radius fracture.

Finally, the role for patient preference must also be considered when selecting operative or nonoperative treatment of distal radius fractures. Patient's preference regarding autonomy, return to daily routines, pain control, ultimate function, and exposure to anesthesia all are cited as considerations when selecting operative or nonoperative treatment.[20] In many cases, patients indicate a preference for internal fixation, when compared with alternative means of operative stabilization.[20] For surgeons interested in a more formal, structured manner to consider patient preference in the treatment of distal radius fractures, point-of-care tools are available for use.[21]

SELECTING THE "RIGHT CARE"
Considerations for Operative Management

AAOS clinical practice guidelines published in 2010 provide the initial framework for the management of distal radius fractures.[14] Specifically, fractures with radial shortening greater than 3 mm, dorsal tilt greater than 10°, or intra-articular displacement greater than 2 mm (**Fig. 1**) following closed reduction should be considered for surgical fixation to optimize pain, function, and complications based on numerous randomized clinical trials.[22–24]

For nonoperative treatment, rigid immobilization is recommended, whereas removable splints in minimally displaced distal radius fractures are considered acceptable practice.[14] Despite the paucity of literature available to further direct treatment based on patient age or specific fracture-morphology,[14] practice patterns of surgeons typically adhere to these basic tenets.[16]

Underlying the recommendation for operative intervention for excessive dorsal tilt or radial shortening is the association between these radiographic measures and functional outcomes (eg, wrist flexion, pinch strength, and ability to perform activities of daily living).[25–27] More complex, however, is the role of articular incongruency in long-term outcomes following distal radius fracture. Goldfarb and colleagues[5] demonstrated the association between residual articular displacement and progressive radiocarpal arthrosis 15 years following injury in a younger patient population. Despite such arthrosis, functional status remained high and was not associated with the degree of arthrosis demonstrated by three-dimensional imaging.[5] Forward and colleagues[6] similarly demonstrated that radiographically apparent post-traumatic arthritis is not associated with functional impairment. Unlike the weight-bearing lower extremity,[28] where articular incongruity leads to symptomatic arthrosis, articular incongruity and

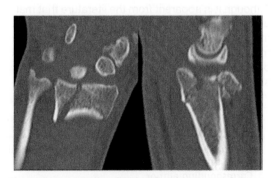

Fig. 1. Intra-articular distal radius fracture with 5 mm of articular incongruity, as demonstrated by preoperative computed tomography scan.

resultant arthrosis does not necessarily portend an individual to unfavorable clinical outcomes following distal radius fracture. Despite the demonstrated lack of association between radiographic arthritis and associated symptoms, many surgeons adhere to the original recommendations of Knirk and Jupiter[29] to minimize articular incongruity of the distal radius, particularly in the younger patient population.

Although LaFontaine criteria of age greater than 60 years, greater than 20° of dorsal angulation, presence of dorsal comminution, intra-articular involvement, and associated ulna fractures are classically used to stratify the risk of secondary displacement,[30] subsequent evaluation of these criteria showed that age is the only significant predictor of displacement.[10] Moreover, based on work by LaMartina and colleagues,[31] the absence of a volar hook (the lack of volar cortex integrity) on postreduction radiographs is associated with increased risk of secondary displacement and subsequent malunion. Although radiographic findings concerning for secondary displacement do not represent a firm indication for operative intervention, such factors are essential to inform patient counseling and follow-up.

The radiographic parameter most useful to the senior author is the position of the capitate relative to the radial shaft on the lateral view (**Fig. 2**), because failure to restore carpal alignment in the sagittal plane has a negative impact on patient-reported functional outcomes.[32] Carpal malalignment is present when the center of the capitate is not aligned with the radial shaft. This is most often seen in dorsally displaced fractures (presumably with dorsal tilt of the radius), but volar displacement of the carpus can also be seen in volar lunate facet fractures. Given the implications that carpal malalignment has for functional outcomes, the presence of carpal malalignment is typically an indication for operative intervention in younger patients.

In our practice, additional consideration is given to radially displaced (coronally shifted) metaphyseal fractures, which have been shown to result in increased distal radioulnar joint (DRUJ) instability (**Fig. 3**)[33,34] because of decreased tension of the distal oblique bundle of the interosseous membrane.[34] Because biomechanical study has demonstrated anatomic reduction of a coronally shifted distal radius fracture restores tension of the distal oblique bundle and improves DRUJ stability, restoration of coronal alignment should be considered during treatment of distal radius fractures.[34,35]

In summary, patients with displaced fractures with carpal malalignment are at highest risk for

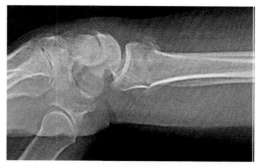

Fig. 2. Extra-articular distal radius fracture with dorsal displacement of the capitate, relative to the radial shaft.

functional compromise. Older patients and those without a restored volar hook after reduction are at risk for displacement and subsequent malalignment. In our practice, most patients with maintained carpal alignment on the lateral view are treated nonoperatively, even if articular incongruity and radial shortening are present. Exceptions are considered based on patient preferences, as described next.

Nonoperative Management

In the setting of minimally displaced distal radius fractures, prospective trials have demonstrated no significant difference between cast and splint

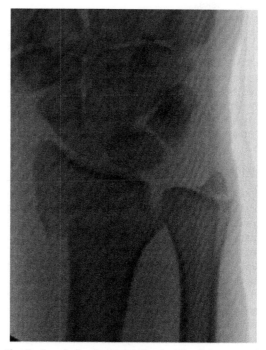

Fig. 3. A radially displaced distal radius fracture with associated ulnar styloid fracture.

immobilization.[36] As such, AAOS guidelines deem the use of removal wrist splints as an acceptable option for immobilization in nondisplaced radius fractures.[14] As such, we offer both methods of immobilization to patients presenting with nondisplaced and minimally displaced distal radius fractures. For individuals choosing to undergo prefabricated splint immobilizations, the patient is always instructed to wear the removal splint except to perform personal hygiene. In most cases, the provision of two removable splints is ideal, to allow the patient to alternate and wash the splints while maintaining appropriate wear. A therapy-fabricated custom orthosis is preferred by some patients but entails increased cost of care.

If a patient with displaced metaphyseal distal radius fracture presents to a facility with the appropriate capability, a closed reduction is performed with conscious sedation or analgesia with an associated hematoma block.[12] Although above-elbow[12] and below-elbow[37,38] immobilization methods have been demonstrated to maintain fracture reduction, we prefer a molded sugar tong splint to maintain postreduction alignment. Following closed reduction and immobilization, patients should be followed closely with serial radiographs[12] to evaluate for subsequent displacement. Nesbitt and colleagues[10] demonstrated that the likelihood of subsequent fracture displacement decreases substantially after the first 2 weeks.

We counsel all patients undergoing nonoperative treatment about the risk of spontaneous extensor pollicis longus rupture. For those patients with notable dorsal displacement and shortening, we describe the expected appearance of the wrist after the expectant malunion. Although the functional result is tolerable, the relative dorsal prominence of the ulnar head is surprising (and off-putting, if unexpected) to some patients.

Method of Operative Fixation

Operative intervention for distal radius fractures in increasingly common, with volar locking plating systems (VLPS) representing the most common method for operative intervention, when compared with percutaneous pinning or external fixation.[39] However, based on data available at the time, AAOS guidelines are unable to identify a superior method for operative fixation.[14] More recently, large, randomized trials demonstrate similar complication rates between methods of operative fixation,[8] although the complication profile of each treatment modality is unique to each technique.

In a large, multicenter, randomized trial performed by Chung and colleagues,[8] internal fixation, external fixation, and closed reduction and pin fixation demonstrated similar 12-month outcomes in patients older than 60 years of age. Such data mirror numerous studies indicating volar plating, external fixation, and pin-fixation all yield similar, acceptable functional outcomes at long-term follow-up.[40–42] However, short-term functional outcomes demonstrate improved early clinical outcomes with volar plate fixation, when compared with nonoperative management[8] and alternative fracture fixation.[8,41] Given the relative ease of a volar approach and application of a volar plate, favorable short-term outcomes associated with VLPS, and similar long-term outcomes across all methods of fracture fixation, standard volar plate fixation represents the preferred treatment modality for most (85%) practicing hand surgeons.[43]

In our practice, the role for external fixation or closed reduction and percutaneous pinning is limited, given the favorable short- and long-term outcomes associated with VLPS. External fixation may be considered in the setting of open and/or grossly contaminated fractures as either definitive fixation or as a temporizing measure before definitive debridement and internal fixation, yet immediate open reduction and internal fixation of open fractures yields satisfactory outcomes.[44] Additionally, external fixation is considered in the setting of severely comminuted, intra-articular fractures that are not amenable to VLPS or fragment-specific fixation. However, dorsal spanning bridge plate fixation has been shown to yield acceptable outcomes in this setting[45] and serves as the preferable option in many cases. Moreover, dorsal bridge plating demonstrated a significantly lower infection rate (2% vs 10%) than external fixation, further supporting this treatment modality.[46]

Although VLPS represents that mainstay of internal fixation, this technique is associated with two mechanisms of suboptimal outcomes: tendon irritation/rupture and loss of fixation. Flexor tendon irritation, particularly when the volar plate is placed distal to the pronator fossa (the watershed line),[47] or flexor pollicis longus tendon rupture occur in approximately 10% of individuals undergoing fixation with a VLPS.[48] Although repair of the pronator quadratus over the volar plate offers the theoretic advantage of reducing flexor pollicis longus contact with the volar plate, prospective studies demonstrate routine repair does not improve functional outcomes or reoperation rates.[49] As such, emphasis on volar plate position relative to the pronator fossa and a low threshold for hardware removal (which occurs in 9% of cases) are paramount.[50] Additionally, extensor pollicis longus and extensor tendon rupture may occur, and is largely attributed to either drill-bit penetration or prominent dorsal screw tips.[51] Yet, with biomechanical study by Wall and colleagues[52] demonstrating that abutment of the volar locking screw to the dorsal cortex is unnecessary for optimal biomechanical strength, dorsal tendon irritation may be largely avoided. Methods to improve fixation into the distal fracture fragment, through moving the volar plate distally or increased locking screw length, may be performed at the risk of increasing tendon irritation.

Loss of fixation commonly occurs with loss of volar tilt or loss of intermediate column fixation. Loss of volar tilt is most likely to occur in instances of significant dorsal comminution, whereby suboptimal locking screw purchase is obtained in the distal fragment.[53] As discussed, the volar locking screws should traverse at least 75% of the radius to provide sufficient biomechanical strength.[52] An advantage of the precontoured volar locking plate is the ability to use the volar plate as a reduction aid during operative intervention. However, attempting to pull the fracture fragment volarly with the plate, rather than apply manual pressure to the dorsal radius to restore volar tilt, may result in inadvertent screw pull-out and loss of reduction (particularly in patients with osteoporosis).

Fragment-specific fixation offers the theoretic benefit of obtaining and maintaining reduction of distal or small fracture fragments: volar ulnar corner fragments, articular shear fragments, central impaction fractures, and dorsal ulnar fragments.[53] Of particular importance is the volar ulnar corner, both the keystone of the articular surface for the radiocarpal and DRUJ and the attachment site for the short radiolunate ligament,[54] which must be reduced to prevent subsequent radiocarpal subluxation.[54] Using a volar buttress plate (with or without a hook), a form of fragment-specific fixation, to address this "critical corner" reliably yields favorable radiographic outcomes,[55] which may be unobtainable through VPLS. In a similar fashion, large radial styloid fragments, containing the insertion of the deforming brachioradialis, may be inadequately fixed with a single volar plate. Moreover, screw placement into the radial styloid may be made difficult by requisite locking screw trajectory and such screws may be prominent within the plate, resulting in flexor tendon irritation. In this case, a contoured radial column plate may more-optimally buttress the radial styloid fragment and prevent placement of prominent locking screws. Although the authors advocate for the use of fragment-specific fixation in certain fracture patterns,[53] available literature has not demonstrated superior outcomes with fragment-specific fixation, when compared with VLPS.[56]

RIGHT TIME

Management of distal radius fractures, whether treated operatively or nonoperatively, must weigh the benefit of early mobilization on ultimate wrist function with the risk of secondary displacement, hardware failure, or wound complication that may occur with premature discontinuation of splint or cast immobilization.

For nondisplaced distal radius fractures, no difference is noted between immobilization for 3 or 5 weeks with a plaster splint.[57] However, given the consensus that plaster immobilization may be unnecessary in this fracture pattern,[14] shorter durations of immobilization followed by bracing is also appropriate. A relative paucity of literature exists to guide the duration of immobilization for displaced distal radius fractures. Generally, cast immobilization for 6 weeks is considered sufficient to allow for adequate callous formation. At this interval, radiographs out of the cast and the clinical absence of tenderness about the fracture site serve as indicators that adequate healing has occurred. In most cases, cast immobilization is transitioned to a removal wrist splint at this juncture. The removable splint is weaned over 2 weeks but may be intermittently used with high-demand activity.

Length of immobilization following VLPS fixation for distal radius fractures varies significantly between surgeons, with surgeon preference ranging between no immobilization and immobilization for 6 weeks.[43] Early motion following VLPS fixation of distal radius fractures has yielded variable outcomes when compared with splint immobilization in the postoperative period.[58,59] Yet, high-level evidence indicates such early mobilization may provide improved short-term range of motion and grip strength.[59] For surgeons choosing to immobilize the arm following volar-plating of the distal radius in the immediate postoperative period, no difference is noted in range of motion, strength, or patient-reported outcomes.[60] Consequently, allowing range of motion and early mobilization immediately following volar plating or brief immobilization in the postoperative period represent acceptable options. As such, it is our preference to immobilize the wrist for 10 to 14 days. After suture removal, early active motion is started. Typically at 4 to 6 weeks after surgery, strengthening is added.

RIGHT COST

Given the frequency of distal radius fractures and the rate of internal fixation, the cost associated with management of these injuries becomes a substantial consideration from a health systems perspective. Specifically, Medicare alone was calculated to spent $170 million on the treatment of distal radius fractures in 2007, with total costs estimated to increase with higher rates of operative intervention.[61] Although the Medicare payment per beneficiary was highest for those individuals treated with internal fixation, most ($92 million) Medicare spending is related to closed treatment.[61] Yet, the cost of isolated distal radius fractures extends beyond the clinic, with 4.4% of patients requiring hospitalization and 20% of hospitalized patients requiring postacute rehabilitation.[62] As such, the episode-based cost of fracture treatment underestimated the direct and indirect cost associated with this injury.

On average, the cost associated with closed treatment of a distal radius fracture is significantly less than the cost of operative management.[61] Yet, when considering the expedited recovery provided by internal fixation, economic analysis indicates operative fixation possess favorable cost-utility when compared with closed treatment in elderly patients.[63] Although most patients are insulated from the cost-differential between treatment modalities (ie, possesses a similar copay regardless of treatment modality), the increase in individual financial responsibility with newer health insurance plans may play an increasing role in patient decision-making.

The direct cost for an episode of care related to internal fixation ($8464) is higher than the cost of either external fixation ($7994) or closed reduction and percutaneous pinning ($5600). Predictably, most cost differential is attributed to the higher surgical cost associated with internal fixation ($6289), when compared with external fixation ($5063) or closed reduction and percutaneous pinning ($3440).[9] However, when considering potential complications and outcomes associated with these methods of operative fixation, internal fixation again provides favorable cost-utility when compared with alternative operative treatments.[63]

In addition to variation between the cost associated with various treatment modalities, significant cost variation exists between cases of distal radius fractures undergoing open reduction an internal fixation.[64] The most significant factor impacting the cost of distal radius fractures is the implant used in operative fixation, with accounts for 48% of total direct cost.[64] Additionally, the cost of such implants can vary widely, with some implants costing three times more than a comparable alternative.[65] Despite most surgeons agreeing implant cost should be factored into device selection, attending physicians correctly estimate the actual

cost of a device only 20% of the time.[66] Given the cost for operative fixation of distal radius fractures is largely driven by the implant, surgeon awareness of cost is essential for providing value-based care.

Another significant portion of the total cost associated with distal radius fractures (38% of total direct cost) is related to the facility where operative intervention is performed.[64] Fractures treated in ambulatory surgery centers are performed at a significantly lower cost than those performed in the inpatient setting, with anesthesia costs ($784 ambulatory vs $909 inpatient), operating room cost ($1827 ambulatory vs $2992 inpatient), and recovery room cost ($295 ambulatory vs $660 inpatient) all favoring treatment in the ambulatory setting, when possible.[67]

Large meta-analysis regarding the clinical benefit of routine physical and occupational therapy is of unclear clinical benefit.[68] Despite this unclear clinical benefit, more than 25% of individuals receive either physical or occupational therapy following operative intervention for a distal radius fracture.[69] Additionally, the total cost of therapy following distal radius fractures is higher than many common hand procedures, such as carpometacarpal arthroplasty, carpal tunnel release, trigger finger release, and ganglion cyst removal. Given the significant cost and unclear benefit, the judicious use of therapy referrals remains a further opportunity for providing care at the optimal cost.

Distal radius fracture sustained from ground-level falls also represent an osteoporosis-defining fracture,[70] therefore warranting evaluation of bone mineral density and initiation of calcium, vitamin D, and/or bisphosphonate therapy. Although the risk of sustaining a second fragility fracture (lumbar compression, proximal humerus, hip fracture) within the next 5 years is significant (approximately 10%), the rate of diagnosis and management of osteoporosis in this population remains suboptimal.[71] Because osteoporotic fractures of the hip are associated with a significant 1-year mortality rate (33%),[72] and bisphosphonate therapy is associated with a decreased mortality rate in patients with osteoporosis,[73] it is incumbent on the upper extremity surgeon to ensure appropriate evaluation and management of these injuries. In secondary prevention, initiation of bisphosphonate therapy represents a highly cost-effective intervention.[74]

Although internal fixation results in the highest episode cost, the improved function and expedited recovery may provide value in the appropriate patient scenario. The surgeon must remain cognizant of cost, particularly as it relates to implant selection, because implant costs represents the most significant driver of total direct cost. Additionally, performing operative intervention in an ambulatory setting when possible represents another significant opportunity to improve the relative value of surgical intervention. After the procedure is performed, the judicious use of therapy referrals and improved recognition of osteoporosis are required to provide cost-effective care.

SUMMARY

The relative frequency of distal radius fractures and the myriad techniques available to manage these injuries requires thorough understanding of the natural history of the untreated disease and impact of intervention on ultimate outcomes to select the appropriate treatment for each patient. For extra-articular distal radius fractures, traditional radiographic measures of radial height and volar tilt are considered given the impact of these measures on physical function. Additional characteristics regarding risk of subsequent displacement, coronal shift impacting DRUJ stability, and carpal alignment should also be considered when selecting ideal treatment. Of these, particular emphasis is placed on carpal alignment in our practice. Finally, articular incongruity, known to lead to the progression of radiocarpal and DRUJ arthrosis, warrants operative intervention, although anatomic reduction may not significantly impact physical function or clinical outcome.[5] For operatively managed fractures, open reduction and internal fixation is the most common treatment modality and may be associated with an expedited recovery at a higher cost than other treatment modalities.

Patient-specific factors, most specifically physiologic age, must be considered when caring for distal radius fractures. Additionally, patient desiring or requiring an expedited return to work or sport may also benefit from internal fixation, regardless of degree of displacement. Moreover, the multiply injured patient may benefit from early improved function allowed by internal fixation.

For patients undergoing nonoperative management, rigid immobilization in a cast or splint for 6 weeks remains the standard treatment. However, treatment in a removable wrist brace is considered for nondisplaced fractures. For patients undergoing internal fixation, early mobilization provides improved range of motion and function in the short term. For this reason, operatively managed distal radius fractures should typically undergo immobilization for 2 weeks or less to protect the surgical incision.

Given the frequency of this injury pattern, optimal management of distal radius must consider the value of each treatment provided. In general, internal fixation represents the most expensive treatment modality, with cost primarily driven by the surgical implant and facility costs. To manage surgical cost, the surgeon may remain cognizant of variations in implant price and preferentially perform surgery in an ambulatory setting. Despite the cost associated with internal fixation, the treatment modality remains cost-effective given the expedited return of function. Further cost-conscious care may be provided through the judicious use of therapy services and appropriate prevention of further fragility fractures.

Through the synthesis of these elements, the optimal treatment for each patient may be selected. Further research is required to better define which patients and what fracture morphologies may benefit from operative intervention. Moreover, the role of newer-generation volar plating systems and fragment-specific fixation technology may alter the relative benefit of operative intervention. In this way, the upper extremity surgeon may continue to better define how to provide the right care to the right patient, at the right time, for the right cost.

CLINICS CARE POINTS

- When performing an initial evaluation of a patient with a displaced distal radius fracture, surgeons should consider the patient- and injury-specific risk factors for symptomatic malunion if the fracture heals in a displaced position.

- Older adults with a distal radius fracture are at high risk for secondary displacement, thus require close clinical follow-up and serial radiographs. The risk for displacement decreases substantially after the first 2 weeks of immobilization.

- When evaluating a lateral radiograph, the most important radiographic parameter is the alignment of the center of the capitate relative to the radial shaft. Dorsal or volar displacement of the carpus relative to the radius increases the risk for poor patient-reported outcomes.

- Placement of a volar plate distal to the watershed may lead to flexor tendon irritation or rupture, while inadvertent drill penetration dorsally or prominent screw placement may result in extensor tendon irritation.

- For displaced volar lunate facet fractures, a standard volar locking plate proximal to the watershed line may not provide sufficient fixation to prevent volar subluxation of the carpus. Fragment specific fixation strategies may be particularly in this subset of fractures.

- Because implant cost comprises nearly half of the total direct cost in operative management, surgeons should be judicious and cost conscious about their implant selection.

DISCLOSURES

The authors report no disclosures relevant to this work.

REFERENCES

1. Karl JW, Olson PR, Rosenwasser MP. The epidemiology of upper extremity fractures in the United States, 2009. J Orthop Trauma 2015;29(8):e242–4.
2. Nellans KW, Kowalski E, Chung KC. The epidemiology of distal radius fractures. Hand Clin 2012; 28(2):113–25.
3. Arora R, Lutz M, Deml C, et al. A prospective randomized trial comparing nonoperative treatment with volar locking plate fixation for displaced and unstable distal radial fractures in patients sixty-five years of age and older. J Bone Joint Surg Am 2011;93(23):2146–53.
4. Bartl C, Stengel D, Bruckner T, et al. The treatment of displaced intra-articular distal radius fractures in elderly patients. Dtsch Arztebl Int 2014;111(46): 779–87.
5. Goldfarb CA, Rudzki JR, Catalano LW, et al. Fifteen-year outcome of displaced intra-articular fractures of the distal radius. J Hand Surg Am 2006;31(4):633–9.
6. Forward DP, Davis TR, Sithole JS. Do young patients with malunited fractures of the distal radius inevitably develop symptomatic post-traumatic osteoarthritis? J Bone Joint Surg Br 2008;90(5):629–37.
7. Hammert WC, Calfee RP. Understanding PROMIS. J Hand Surg Am 2020;45(7):650–4.
8. Chung KC, Kim HM, Malay S, et al. The wrist and radius injury surgical trial: 12-month outcomes from a multicenter international randomized clinical trial. Plast Reconstr Surg 2020;145(6):1054e–66e.
9. Huetteman HE, Zhong L, Chung KC. Cost of surgical treatment for distal radius fractures and the implications of episode-based bundled payments. J Hand Surg Am 2018;43(8):720–30.
10. Nesbitt KS, Failla JM, Les C. Assessment of instability factors in adult distal radius fractures. J Hand Surg Am 2004;29(6):1128–38.
11. Makhni EC, Ewald TJ, Kelly S, et al. Effect of patient age on the radiographic outcomes of distal radius fractures subject to nonoperative treatment. J Hand Surg Am 2008;33(8):1301–8.
12. Levin LS, Rozell JC, Pulos N. Distal radius fractures in the elderly. J Am Acad Orthop Surg 2017;25(3): 179–87.
13. Nelson GN, Stepan JG, Osei DA, et al. The impact of patient activity level on wrist disability after distal radius malunion in older adults. J Orthop Trauma 2015;29(4):195–200.
14. Lichtman DM, Bindra RR, Boyer MI, et al. Treatment of distal radius fractures. J Am Acad Orthop Surg 2010;18(3):180–9.
15. Ochen Y, Peek J, van der Velde D, et al. Operative vs nonoperative treatment of distal radius fractures in adults: a systematic review and meta-analysis. JAMA Netw Open 2020;3(4):e203497.
16. Okoroafor UC, Cannada LK. Do orthopedic trauma surgeons adhere to AAOS guidelines when treating distal radius fractures? Iowa Orthop J 2018;38: 53–60.
17. MacFarlane RJ, Miller D, Wilson L, et al. Functional outcome and complications at 2.5 years following volar locking plate fixation of distal radius fractures. J Hand Microsurg 2015;7(1):18–24.
18. Beleckas C, Calfee R. Distal radius fractures in the athlete. Curr Rev Musculoskelet Med 2017;10(1): 62–71.
19. Kang SW, Shin WC, Moon NH, et al. Concomitant hip and upper extremity fracture in elderly patients: prevalence and clinical implications. Injury 2019; 50(11):2045–8.
20. Nasser JS, Huetteman HE, Shauver MJ, et al. Older patient preferences for internal fixation after a distal radius fracture: a qualitative study from the wrist and radius injury surgical trial. Plast Reconstr Surg 2018; 142(1):34e–41e.
21. Shapiro LM, Eppler SL, Baker LC, et al. The usability and feasibility of conjoint analysis to elicit preferences for distal radius fractures in patients 55 years and older. J Hand Surg Am 2019;44(10):846–52.
22. Young CF, Nanu AM, Checketts RG. Seven-year outcome following Colles' type distal radial fracture. A comparison of two treatment methods. J Hand Surg Br 2003;28(5):422–6.
23. Abbaszadegan H, Jonsson U. External fixation or plaster cast for severely displaced Colles' fractures? Prospective 1-year study of 46 patients. Acta Orthop Scand 1990;61(6):528–30.
24. Pring DJ, Barber L, Williams DJ. Bipolar fixation of fractures of the distal end of the radius: a comparative study. Injury 1988;19(3):145–8.
25. Plant CE, Parsons NR, Costa ML. Do radiological and functional outcomes correlate for fractures of the distal radius? Bone Joint J 2017;99-b(3):376–82.
26. McQueen M, Caspers J. Colles fracture: does the anatomical result affect the final function? J Bone Joint Surg Br 1988;70(4):649–51.

27. Villar RN, Marsh D, Rushton N, et al. Three years after Colles' fracture. A prospective review. J Bone Joint Surg Br 1987;69(4):635–8.

28. Clarke-Jenssen J, Wikerøy AKB, Røise O, et al. Long-term survival of the native hip after a minimally displaced, nonoperatively treated acetabular fracture. J Bone Joint Surg Am 2016;98(16):1392–9.

29. Knirk JL, Jupiter JB. Intra-articular fractures of the distal end of the radius in young adults. J Bone Joint Surg Am 1986;68(5):647–59.

30. Lafontaine M, Hardy D, Delince P. Stability assessment of distal radius fractures. Injury 1989;20(4):208–10.

31. LaMartina J, Jawa A, Stucken C, et al. Predicting alignment after closed reduction and casting of distal radius fractures. J Hand Surg Am 2015;40(5):934–9.

32. McQueen MM, Hajducka C, Court-Brown CM. Redisplaced unstable fractures of the distal radius: a prospective randomised comparison of four methods of treatment. J Bone Joint Surg Br 1996;78(3):404–9.

33. Kloss JG, Clawson MC. Commentary regarding "The impact of coronal alignment on distal radioulnar joint stability following distal radius fracture. J Hand Surg Am 2014;39(7):1273.

34. Dy CJ, Jang E, Taylor SA, et al. The impact of coronal alignment on distal radioulnar joint stability following distal radius fracture. J Hand Surg Am 2014;39(7):1264–72.

35. Trehan SK, Orbay JL, Wolfe SW. Coronal shift of distal radius fractures: influence of the distal interosseous membrane on distal radioulnar joint instability. J Hand Surg Am 2015;40(1):159–62.

36. Tumia N, Wardlaw D, Hallett J, et al. Aberdeen Colles' fracture brace as a treatment for Colles' fracture. A multicentre, prospective, randomised, controlled trial. J Bone Joint Surg Br 2003;85(1):78–82.

37. Jackson T, Maulsby E, Wilson D, et al. A comparison of sugar-tong and volar-dorsal splints for provisional immobilization of distal radius fractures in the adult population. Eur J Orthop Surg Traumatol 2020. https://doi.org/10.1007/s00590-020-02760-w.

38. Maluta T, Dib G, Cengarle M, et al. Below- vs above-elbow cast for distal radius fractures: is elbow immobilization really effective for reduction maintenance? Int Orthop 2019;43(10):2391–7.

39. Chung KC, Shauver MJ, Birkmeyer JD. Trends in the United States in the treatment of distal radial fractures in the elderly. J Bone Joint Surg Am 2009;91(8):1868–73.

40. Franceschi F, Franceschetti E, Paciotti M, et al. Volar locking plates versus K-wire/pin fixation for the treatment of distal radial fractures: a systematic review and quantitative synthesis. Br Med Bull 2015;115(1):91–110.

41. Zhou Y, Zhu Y, Zhang X, et al. Comparison of radiographic and functional results of die-punch fracture of distal radius between volar locking plating (VLP) and external fixation (EF). J Orthop Surg Res 2019;14(1):373.

42. Williksen JH, Husby T, Hellund JC, et al. External fixation and adjuvant pins versus volar locking plate fixation in unstable distal radius fractures: a randomized, controlled study with a 5-year follow-up. J Hand Surg Am 2015;40(7):1333–40.

43. Salibian AA, Bruckman KC, Bekisz JM, et al. Management of unstable distal radius fractures: a survey of hand surgeons. J Wrist Surg 2019;8(4):335–43.

44. Harper CM, Dowlatshahi AS, Rozental TD. Evaluating outcomes following open fractures of the distal radius. J Hand Surg Am 2020;45(1):41–7.

45. Lauder A, Agnew S, Bakri K, et al. Functional outcomes following bridge plate fixation for distal radius fractures. J Hand Surg Am 2015;40(8):1554–62.

46. Wang WL, Ilyas AM. Dorsal bridge plating versus external fixation for distal radius fractures. J Wrist Surg 2020;9(2):177–84.

47. Orbay J. Volar plate fixation of distal radius fractures. Hand Clin 2005;21(3):347–54.

48. Arora R, Lutz M, Hennerbichler A, et al. Complications following internal fixation of unstable distal radius fracture with a palmar locking-plate. J Orthop Trauma 2007;21(5):316–22.

49. Tosti R, Ilyas AM. Prospective evaluation of pronator quadratus repair following volar plate fixation of distal radius fractures. J Hand Surg Am 2013;38(9):1678–84.

50. Yamamoto M, Fujihara Y, Fujihara N, et al. A systematic review of volar locking plate removal after distal radius fracture. Injury 2017;48(12):2650–6.

51. Berglund LM, Messer TM. Complications of volar plate fixation for managing distal radius fractures. J Am Acad Orthop Surg 2009;17(6):369–77.

52. Wall LB, Brodt MD, Silva MJ, et al. The effects of screw length on stability of simulated osteoporotic distal radius fractures fixed with volar locking plates. J Hand Surg Am 2012;37(3):446–53.

53. Dy CJ, Wolfe SW, Jupiter JB, et al. Distal radius fractures: strategic alternatives to volar plate fixation. Instr Course Lect 2014;63:27–37.

54. O'Shaughnessy MA, Shin AY, Kakar S. Stabilization of volar ulnar rim fractures of the distal radius: current techniques and review of the literature. J Wrist Surg 2016;5(2):113–9.

55. Biondi M, Keller M, Merenghi L, et al. Hook plate for volar rim fractures of the distal radius: review of the first 23 cases and focus on dorsal radiocarpal dislocation. J Wrist Surg 2019;8(2):93–9.

56. Sammer DM, Fuller DS, Kim HM, et al. A comparative study of fragment-specific versus

volar plate fixation of distal radius fractures. Plast Reconstr Surg 2008;122(5):1441–50.

57. Christensen OM, Christiansen TG, Krasheninnikoff M, et al. Length of immobilisation after fractures of the distal radius. Int Orthop 1995;19(1):26–9.

58. Clementsen S, Hammer OL, Šaltytė Benth J, et al. Early mobilization and physiotherapy vs. late mobilization and home exercises after ORIF of distal radial fractures: a randomized controlled trial. JB JS Open Access 2019;4(3). https://doi.org/10.2106/jbjs.oa.19.00012.

59. Quadlbauer S, Pezzei C, Jurkowitsch J, et al. Early rehabilitation of distal radius fractures stabilized by volar locking plate: a prospective randomized pilot study. J Wrist Surg 2017;6(2):102–12.

60. Hill JR, Navo PD, Bouz G, et al. Immobilization following distal radius fractures: a randomized clinical trial. J Wrist Surg 2018;7(5):409–14.

61. Shauver MJ, Yin H, Banerjee M, et al. Current and future national costs to Medicare for the treatment of distal radius fracture in the elderly. J Hand Surg Am 2011;36(8):1282–7.

62. Zhong L, Mahmoudi E, Giladi AM, et al. Utilization of post-acute care following distal radius fracture among Medicare beneficiaries. J Hand Surg Am 2015;40(12):2401–9.e8.

63. Shauver MJ, Clapham PJ, Chung KC. An economic analysis of outcomes and complications of treating distal radius fractures in the elderly. J Hand Surg Am 2011;36(12):1912–8.e1-3.

64. Kazmers NH, Judson CH, Presson AP, et al. Evaluation of factors driving cost variation for distal radius fracture open reduction internal fixation. J Hand Surg Am 2018;43(7):606–14.e1.

65. Beredjiklian PK. Shelf pricing for distal radius fracture implants. Clin Orthop Relat Res 2017;475(3):595–6.

66. Okike K, O'Toole RV, Pollak AN, et al. Survey finds few orthopedic surgeons know the costs of the devices they implant. Health Aff (Millwood) 2014;33(1):103–9.

67. Mather RC 3rd, Wysocki RW, Mack Aldridge J 3rd, et al. Effect of facility on the operative costs of distal radius fractures. J Hand Surg Am 2011;36(7):1142–8.

68. Handoll HH, Elliott J. Rehabilitation for distal radial fractures in adults. Cochrane Database Syst Rev 2015;(9):Cd003324.

69. Shah RF, Zhang S, Li K, et al. Physical and occupational therapy use and cost after common hand procedures. J Hand Surg Am 2020;45(4):289–97.e1.

70. Lorentzon M, Cummings SR. Osteoporosis: the evolution of a diagnosis. J Intern Med 2015;277(6):650–61.

71. Benzvi L, Gershon A, Lavi I, et al. Secondary prevention of osteoporosis following fragility fractures of the distal radius in a large health maintenance organization. Arch Osteoporos 2016;11:20.

72. Guzon-Illescas O, Perez Fernandez E, Crespí Villarias N, et al. Mortality after osteoporotic hip fracture: incidence, trends, and associated factors. J Orthop Surg Res 2019;14(1):203.

73. Bliuc D, Tran T, van Geel T, et al. Mortality risk reduction differs according to bisphosphonate class: a 15-year observational study. Osteoporos Int 2019;30(4):817–28.

74. Akehurst R, Brereton N, Ariely R, et al. The cost effectiveness of zoledronic acid 5 mg for the management of postmenopausal osteoporosis in women with prior fractures: evidence from Finland, Norway and the Netherlands. J Med Econ 2011;14(1):53–64.

Outcome Measurement for Distal Radius Fractures

Matthew J. Hall, MD[a], Peter J. Ostergaard, MD[a], Tamara D. Rozental, MD[b],*

KEYWORDS

- Distal radius fracture • Standardized outcome measurement • Value-based health care delivery
- Patient-reported outcome measure

KEY POINTS

- Standardized patient outcomes enable comparisons among health care services and are an important step in the implementation of value-based health care.
- A standardized patient outcome instrument for distal radius fractures should include assessment of pain, a validated patient-reported outcome scale, performance measures, radiographs, and an assessment of complications.
- Patient-specific and injury-specific factors that modify outcomes should be adjusted.
- Outcomes should follow along a standardized timeline with the use of electronic adjuncts to decrease the burden to patients, providers, and researchers.

IMPORTANCE OF DEFINING OUTCOMES FOR DISTAL RADIUS FRACTURES

Distal radius fractures (DRFs) are among the most common upper extremity injuries in adults and the second most common fracture in the elderly population.[1–4] The incidence of these fractures is increasing, and a greater proportion are being treated with open reduction internal fixation (ORIF).[1,5–7] Although preliminary studies have shown that ORIF is a financially viable solution, the economic burden of this injury clearly is increasing.[2,7–9] In the context of increasing health care expenditures, some economists have proposed restructuring payments to a value-based health care delivery system.[10,11] The basis of a value-based care system relies on the definition of value as health outcomes achieved divided by dollars spent.[12] Transitioning to a value-based system requires standardization of outcomes to allow meaningful comparison across varying health care systems.[4,13] Despite growing interest in the research of DRFs, there currently is no standardized approach to measure outcomes after these

injuries.[4] Furthermore, multiple systematic reviews report outcome heterogeneity limits conclusions.[14–18] Hand surgery does not fit into the traditional surgical outcomes framework given the low associated mortality but large impact on quality of life.[19] Preliminary steps toward standardized outcomes was promoted by a 2009 DRF working group that established a conceptual framework and identified key domains for measurements.[14] Subsequent research has built on these recommendations, summarizing performance measures, radiographic outcomes, patient-reported outcome measures (PROMs), and complications.[4] This article reviews established recommendations for outcome measures and the next steps, including the International Consortium for Health Outcomes Measurement (ICHOM) development of standardized outcome sets.

STEPS TOWARD CONSENSUS OUTCOMES

Outcome measurement for DRFs has evolved over time. Early instruments, such as the Gartland and Werley score, Green and O'Brien score, and

[a] Harvard Combined Orthopaedic Residency Program, 55 Fruit Street, Boston, MA 02114, USA; [b] Division of Hand and Upper Extremity Surgery, Department of Orthopedics, Beth Israel Deaconess Medical Center, Harvard Medical School, 330 Brookline Avenue, Stoneman 10, Boston, MA 02115, USA
* Corresponding author.
E-mail address: trozenta@bidmc.harvard.edu

Hand Clin 37 (2021) 215–227
https://doi.org/10.1016/j.hcl.2021.02.004

Mayo wrist score, placed an emphasis on pain; performance measures, such as range of motion (ROM) and grip strength; and radiographic outcomes.[20–24] Recently, there has been an increasing interest in PROMs. Over the past few years, several groups have attempted to compare outcomes following DRFs.[25–27] A significant step in standardized outcomes occurred with the organization of a Distal Radius Working Group of the International Society for Fracture Repair and the International Osteoporosis Foundation.[14] From 2009 to 2011, this group of 21 experts, including clinicians, physiotherapists, methodologists, researchers, and industry representatives, determined recommendations on a set of key outcomes following DRFs. This working group used a systematic literature review, nominal group technique, and the World Health Organization International Classification of Functioning, Disability and Health as a conceptual framework.[14] The consensus recommendations of the group were that pain and function should be the 2 primary domains, with complications and return to participation into normal life roles as additional outcomes. For pain measurement, they recommended use of a visual analog scale (VAS), numeric rating scale (NRS), or a specific pain subscale, such as that found in the Patient-Rated Wrist Evaluation (PRWE).[14,28,29] For functional measurement, they recommended PROMs, such as PRWE or Disability of the Arm, Shoulder and Hand (DASH) scale, acknowledging a large degree of overlap between scales.[14] The group emphasized the importance of following complications but acknowledged a lack of standardization, despite preliminary efforts.[30] The group also concluded that shorter outcome scales are more logistically feasible for clinical practice, whereas longer versions of outcome scales may add more granularity for research. A 2016 review by the Distal Radius Outcomes Consortium built on these preliminary recommendations by reviewing several PROMs as well as other outcomes, such as radiographic measurements, coping strategies, and performance-based tests (ROM and grip strength).[4] This group also suggested that timing of outcome measurements should be standardized and patient-specific and injury-specific factors that may have an impact on outcomes should be adjusted for.

PAIN

Pain universally is considered one of the most important outcome measures following DRFs.[4,14] Pain is the predominant symptom in the early recovery period and can lead to greater health care utilization if inadequately controlled.[4,31,32] Although pain is included in several outcome measures, such as DASH, PRWE, Michigan Hand Questionnaire (MHQ), and Patient-Reported Outcomes Measurement Information System (PROMIS), considering only the aggregate score may minimize the importance and impact of pain, which may be the major factor influencing early PROMs.[33,34] For this reason, groups have recommended use of VAS or NRS scales, which specifically examine pain severity and are easily understood.[4,14] Beyond the severity scale, pain assessment should include frequency, qualitative description, and associated/aggravating factors, such as repetitive movements and heavy load bearing.[14] These qualities may be captured efficiently by a validated subscale, such as the DASH, PRWE, MHQ, or PROMIS.[28,33,35–37]

Pain scores should be interpreted in the context of patient-specific and disease-specific factors that may influence outcomes. Injury compensation, patient education, and prereduction radial shortening all have been shown to predict pain response.[38] Furthermore, baseline pain levels predict chronic pain in DRF patients.[32,39] Scoring scales, such as the PROMIS Pain Interference subscale (PROMIS PI), have been developed to measure coping strategies for pain management.[40] Although pain is an established core outcome following DRFs, results should be considered in the context of patient and injury-specific characteristics.

PATIENT-REPORTED OUTCOMES MEASURES

PROMs are powerful tools that convert patients' subjective assessments of symptoms into numeric scores. They quantify the effect of the health condition through symptom severity, activity limitation, and overall impact on quality of life. Furthermore, they are better predictors of return to work and ability to perform activities of daily living (ADLs) than traditional performance measures.[4,41] PROMs increasingly have been emphasized as part of patient-centered care models, and there is evidence that their incorporation may decrease health care utilization and expenditures.[42] Furthermore, these questionnaires are self-administered, require no equipment or examiner, eliminate observer bias, and are easier to perform than physical testing.[26,43]

Several PROMs for upper extremity conditions have been devised, implemented, and validated with different foci ranging from wrist function, to upper extremity function, and to the impact of the upper extremity condition on overall quality of life (**Table 1**).[27] In considering different PROMs

Table 1
Patient-reported outcome tools for upper extremity injuries

Patient-Reported Outcome Measure	Description	Abbreviated Format
PRWE	• 15-item questionnaire • Pain and disability subscales • Designed specifically for conditions affecting the wrist • Reliable, valid, responsive • Established MCID for DRFs	None
DASH	• 30-item questionnaire • Assesses pain and function as it relates to work and activities of daily life • Reliable, valid, responsive • MCID reported, none specific to DRFs • Limited by ceiling effect	QuickDASH • 11-item questionnaire • Abbreviated, validated version of DASH questionnaire • Additional modules for work, sports, performing arts • MCID established for DRFs
MHQ	• 37-item questionnaire • Six domains: pain, overall hand function, ADLs, work performance, aesthetics, satisfaction • Assesses each hand separately • Reliable, valid, responsive • No established MCID for DRFs • Limited by ceiling effect	bMHQ • 12-item questionnaire • Captures same domains as MHQ • Does not assess each hand separately • No established MCID for DRFs
SF-36	• 36-item questionnaire • Eight domains: physical functioning, physical roles, pain, general health, vitality, social functioning, emotional health, mental health • Less responsive than PRWE or DASH • Good validity and reliability for DRFs • No established MCID for DRFs • Places DRFs into context of overall health	SF-12 • 12-item questionnaire • Captures same domains as SF-36 • No established MCID for DRFs
PROMIS UE	• 16-question item bank • Strongly correlates with both DASH and MHQ • Efficient CAT format • No established MCID for DRFs • Limited by ceiling effect and non-normal distribution	None

for DRFs, there is a balance between specificity and breadth. More specific PROMs, such as the PRWE, reveal greater detail about the impact of an injury on a specific area but are less reflective of the injury's impact on the overall health of the individual compared with a more generalized outcome measure, such as the 36-Item Short Form Health Survey (SF-36).[27] Despite multiple comparisons, no PROM has emerged as clearly superior.[25–27]

Patient-Rated Wrist Evaluation

The PRWE is a 15-item questionnaire with sub-scales to measure wrist pain and disability.[28,44] Multiple studies have established the PRWE as a reliable, valid, and responsive tool for DRF outcome measurement.[28,29,45] By design, it is specific for outcome measurement of wrist conditions, which renders it among the most commonly used tools for DRF outcome measurement.[25,27,44] The extensive investigation of the PRWE also includes an established minimal clinically important difference (MCID) of 11.5 points, specifically for DRFs, which assists researchers in determining the clinical relevance of their findings.[46,47] Finally, the PRWE correlates with other well-established PROMs for DRFs, such as the DASH as well as VAS pain scores.[25,48] The main limitation of the PRWE is that its specificity limits generalizability regarding the impact of the injury on the overall health of the individual.[27]

Disabilities of the Arm, Shoulder and Hand and QuickDASH

The DASH is a 30-item tool that measures physical function and symptoms for upper extremity conditions.[36] Beyond the standard assessment of pain and function, the DASH includes additional modules for return to work, sports, and performing arts.[4,36] This system has been extensively studied and proved valid, reliable, and responsive for DRFs.[45,49] It is a less specific instrument than the PRWE, but there is strong correlation between these scales.[27] Several studies have attempted to establish an MCID for the DASH scale (5–15), but there is no MCID specific to DRFs.[50–52] This may limit the interpretation of results by clinicians and researchers. Another limitation to the DASH may be its ceiling effect.[53]

The QuickDASH is an abbreviated format of the DASH and was designed using item-retention techniques to maintain the integrity of the original instrument.[34] Shorter questionnaires take less time to complete, which can improve response rates and quality of data.[34,54–56] The QuickDASH is comparable to its parent DASH scale with the additional benefits of a shorter instrument. Similar to the DASH scale, studies have attempted to establish an MCID for the QuickDASH scale (14–26), including an MCID specific to surgically treated DRFs (26).[51,52]

Michigan Hand Questionnaire and Brief Michigan Hand Questionnaire

The MHQ is a 37-item instrument that measures 6 domains for both upper extremities—pain, overall hand function, activities of daily living, work performance, aesthetics, and satisfaction.[37,57] It is unique among similar outcome instruments in that it measures each hand separately.[4,57,58] Moreover, it is the only upper extremity outcome instrument that incorporates aesthetic considerations.[57] Its psychometric properties are well established, with excellent reliability, validity, responsiveness, and internal consistency.[37,57,59] Although the MHQ MCID has been established for other upper extremity conditions (8–23), an attempt to establish an MCID for DRF patients treated with ORIF was limited by a ceiling effect, because most patients return to a normal high level of function by 3 months postoperatively.[60,61]

Similar to the QuickDASH, an abbreviated scale was developed, the Brief MHQ (bMHQ).[62] The bMHQ covers the same 6 core domains as the MHQ and is similarly valid, reliable, responsive while taking approximately half the time to complete.[57,62] The bMHQ differs from its parent MHQ in that it does not distinguish laterality, but this may be less relevant for DRFs than for bilateral conditions.[62] Similar to the MHQ, no bMHQ MCID has been established for DRFs.

36-Item Short Form Health Survey

The SF-36 is a 36-item instrument that measures health status across 8 domains: physical functioning, physical roles, pain, general health, vitality, social functioning, emotional health, and mental health.[63] The SF-36 was a popular early outcome measurement for DRFs.[26] In comparison to upper extremity–specific outcome scores, the SF-36 evaluates the effect of the injury on the overall health of the individual. This perspective is helpful to capture the impact an upper extremity injury has on overall quality of life. Given the broader scope of the instrument, it is less responsive than its more specific counterparts, such as the DASH and PRWE.[27] Nevertheless, it has well-established validity and reliability throughout the health outcomes literature, including DRF patients, specifically.[26,64,65] The 12-Item Short Form Health Survey (SF-12) is an abbreviated version that carries the advantages of being more concise, correlating well to the SF-36, and being efficacious in the DRF patient population.[55,66–69]

Patient-Reported Outcomes Measurement Information System

The PROMIS was developed by the National Institutes of Health as an integrated instrument to capture self-reported health status across 3 major domains: physical, mental, and social health.[70,71] Within these 3 domains exist subdomains, such as physical function and pain interference within the physical health domain.[71] Item banks are developed for each of these subdomains using computerized adaptive testing (CAT). CAT uses item response theory to estimate level of function and select appropriate items from the bank for testing.[70–74] The advantage of CAT is its ability to achieve greater precision with fewer questions.[72,74,75] Although initial studies showed that the PROMIS Physical Function (PF) CAT compared well to legacy PROMs, additional studies have raised concern about the ceiling effect of this instrument as well as insufficient variance from lower extremity outcome measures.[53,72,76–78] These concerns prompted the development of a distinct 16-item upper extremity subscale (PROMIS UE CAT).[79] Examination of the PROMIS UE CAT has demonstrated that it strongly correlates with the PROMIS PF CAT and other PROMs, such as the QuickDASH and MHQ.[77,80–82] Unfortunately, the PROMIS UE CAT is limited by a non-normal distribution and ceiling effect, with limited ability to distinguish between patients with higher levels of function.[77,80] Although all other PROMIS scales range from 0 to 100 and use a score of 50 as the population normal for easy interpretation, the PROMIS UE CAT does not follow a normal distribution with a high score of 56, creating a ceiling effect that makes higher levels of function difficult to distinguish.[80,82] Despite high correlation, PROMIS UE CAT scores and PROMIS PF CAT scores cannot be compared directly, and PROMIS PF CAT scores are more relevant to compare function across a variety of conditions.[80] Furthermore, PROMIS PF CAT has been studied more extensively and an MCID has been established for DRF patients managed without surgery (3.6–4.6).[83] The PROMIS item bank with CAT administration is an important step toward efficient standardization of outcomes for upper extremity patients. Despite this advance, there are several limitations to the PROMIS UE CAT item bank, including its non-normal score distribution, ceiling effect, and inability to compare the overall impact

of health to other conditions. Further research is needed to refine this instrument.

The PROMIS framework also includes the PROMIS PI CAT, and multiple studies have shown that these scores correlate with the PROMIS functional scales as well as traditional upper extremity PROMs, improving the ability to account for pain interference in the interpretation of functional scores.[72,84]

PATIENT-REPORTED OUTCOME MEASURE LIMITATIONS

Despite advances in the development of PROMs for upper extremity conditions, all of the currently available instruments have limitations. An ideal instrument would demonstrate excellent reliability, validity, and internal consistency, without floor or ceiling effects. It would efficiently achieve a balance between specificity to the condition of interest and relatability to a patient's overall health. Strong correlation with pain-interference measures enables understanding the effects of pain and coping strategies on the overall outcome.[72,84] Establishing condition-specific MCID for each instrument is important, because small improvements may be clinically significant for some conditions. Without condition-specific MCID, clinicians are left to compare these patients to the general population. The traumatic nature of DRFs limits the ability to collect a true baseline functional score for these patients.[57,60,85] Furthermore, many DRF patients return to near-baseline values at 3 months, which reflects both the time course of this injury and a possible limitation of the instrument.[60]

RADIOGRAPHIC OUTCOMES

Radiographs are an essential instrument in DRF management, because they provide information about the injury as well as post-treatment alignment, healing, and hardware position. Traditional outcome measures and their corresponding normal values for alignment include the measurement of radial length (12.3 mm), radial inclination (22o), volar tilt (11o), and ulnar variance (0.4 mm) obtained by posteroanterior and lateral views with the forearm in neutral rotation (**Fig. 1**).[86–88] Multiple studies have attempted to define malunion.[86,89,90] The authors generally follow the parameters reported by Haase and Chung:[86] radial inclination less than 10o, volar tilt greater than 20o or dorsal tilt greater than 20o, radial height less than 10 mm, ulnar variance greater than 2 mm, and intra-articular gap greater than 2 mm. A measurement for assessing radiographic healing

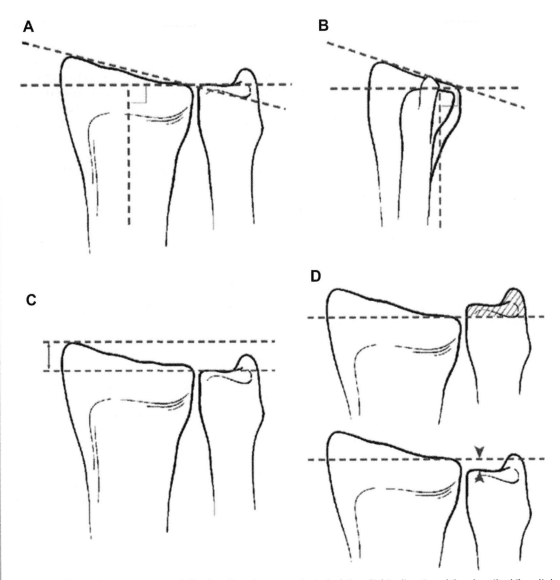

Fig. 1. Radiographic parameters of distal radius alignment include (*A*) radial inclination, (*B*) volar tilt, (*C*) radial height, and (*D*) ulnar variance. (*From* Sharpe F, Stevanovic M. Extra-articular distal radial fracture malunion. Hand Clin 2005;21(3):469–87.)[117]

has been defined for DRFs but this has not been validated.[91] This radiographic union scoring system provides a score of 0 to 2, based on the degree of healing, to each of the 4 cortices on posteroanterior and lateral views of the wrist, for a total score between 0 and 8.[91] Although these parameters are a helpful guide to management, multiple studies have shown that radiographic indices do not correlate with functional outcomes in elderly patients.[17,66,68,92–94] Radiographs are essential in the management of patients with DRFs, providing information that complements parameters, such as pain and PROMs. Despite these benefits, the routine measurement of

radiographic indices should not be considered a primary outcome.

PERFORMANCE MEASURES

Grip strength and ROM of digits, wrist, and forearm traditionally were among the most common outcome measures reported following DRFs.[4,14,16,17] Multiple studies have demonstrated that limited motion through upper extremity joints impairs function and ADLs.[95,96] Grip strength, key pinch, and wrist motion all contribute to patient satisfaction following DRFs.[97] Further research has demonstrated that these performance measures correlate with subjective PROMs.[95,98–100] Among their limitations, PROMs offer a summary score that does not distinguish the contributions of specific items to a patient's sense of disability. Objective performance measures can offer treating surgeons more granular information on the contribution to the patient's sense of disability and thus remain clinically useful. The authors, therefore, recommend goniometer measurement of wrist and forearm ROM and grip strength following DRFs. Grip strength should be measured as a ratio of affected/unaffected extremity to control for variability between patients.[26,27]

COMPLICATIONS

The reported complication rate varies widely in the DRF literature.[30,101–104] Although a standardized checklist has been proposed, this has not been widely adopted.[30] Consensus statements acknowledged a lack of standardization and recommended classifying complications into early and late.[4,14] There also is a range in severity of the complication, because some complications do not influence the patient-perceived disability whereas others require reoperation. For instance, a radiographic malunion in a young patient may cause a functional deficit requiring reoperation, whereas a similar malunion may have no functional consequence in an elderly patient. From a surgeon perspective, it also may be helpful to categorize complications by the tissue they affect, because this may have the greatest impact on treatment. McKay and colleagues[30] proposed the organization of complications by both severity and the tissue type. For instance, malunion or loss of reduction may fall under a skeletal category, carpal tunnel syndrome and complex region pain syndrome under a nerve category, and tendinopathy or tendon rupture under a tendon category. For each complication, there is a grading of severity from mild to severe. A standardized evaluation for the rate and severity of complications is a vital component of any standardized outcome set.

FACTORS THAT MODIFY OUTCOMES

Responsible outcome measurement also accounts for patient-specific and injury-specific characteristics that can alter outcomes. Prior consensus statements recommended classification of these risk factors into sociodemographic, physiologic, psychological, procedural, and injury factors (**Table 2**).[4] Patient-specific factors, such as age, functional demands, and coping

Table 2
Factors having an impact on distal radius fracture patient outcomes

Factor	Examples
Sociodemographic	Age, sex, race, work status, education, occupation, hobbies
Physiologic	Medical comorbidities, preinjury functional level, prior injury, preexisting arthritis
Psychological	Depression, catastrophic thinking, baseline pain level, coping strategies
Injury	Fracture classification, open fracture, nerve injury, ipsilateral extremity fracture
Treatment	Surgical fixation vs closed reduction, time to treatment, type of fixation, occupational therapy

strategies, may influence patient expectations for recovery whereas injury-specific factors, such as fracture classification and associated injuries, also can have an impact on outcome.[32,40,105–110] Psychological factors, such as depression, catastrophic thinking, and baseline pain levels, have been the subject of recent research and are gaining increasing attention for their influence on outcomes.[32,40] The PROMIS PI CAT has demonstrated correlation with upper extremity PROMs and may provide a standardized way of accounting for these variables.[72,84] In order to broadly adopt standardized outcomes, similar accountability must exist for the patient and injury-specific factors that can influence these outcomes.

TIMING OF OUTCOME ASSESSMENTS

Creating comparable outcomes also requires creating a standardized timeline on which to measure outcomes. Several important baseline patient-specific and injury-specific characteristics are collected at the time of injury, such as sociodemographic information and baseline patient characteristics. The use of PROMs with traumatic injuries historically has been limited by inability to obtain a true baseline of function for these patients.[60,85] Although it can be practically

Table 3
Standard outcome assessment timeline

Treatment	Two Weeks	Six Weeks	Twelve Weeks	One Year
ORIF	• Pain (VAS/NRS) • PROM • Radiographs • Complications	• Pain (VAS/NRS) • PROM • ROM, grip strength • Radiographs • Complications	• Pain (VAS/NRS) • PROM • ROM, grip strength • Radiographs • Complications	• Pain (VAS/NRS) • PROM • ROM, grip strength • Radiographs • Complications
Nonoperative management (closed reduction and casting)	• Pain (VAS/NRS) • PROM • Radiographs • Complications	• Pain (VAS/NRS) • PROM • ROM, grip strength • Radiographs • Complications	• Pain (VAS/NRS) • PROM • ROM, grip strength • Radiographs • Complications	• Pain (VAS/NRS) • PROM • ROM, grip strength • Radiographs • Complications

challenging to collect this information at the time of injury, this can offer valuable information regarding an individual's baseline functional status. In the authors' practice, patient outcomes assessment occurs in standardized fashion at 2 weeks, 6 weeks, and 12 weeks after injury and then at 1 year in operatively managed patients.[111] Follow-up at 12 weeks is important because several studies have shown that patients with DRFs regain a significant amount of function by that stage.[26,60,94] Improvements continue for a year, however, leading the authors to believe that longer-term follow-up also should be included to monitor for late complications and final functional evaluation.[4,85] The evolution of electronic medical records and electronic CAT questionnaires may allow for continued long-term follow-up of patients' functional outcomes without significant burden to the patient or provider.[112,113]

SUMMARY

Standardized outcome reporting has enormous potential to reshape health care. A standardized outcome instrument integrates the growing abundance of medical research and permits outcome comparison. Outcome comparison is a step toward the transparency necessary to inform patients and payers in the objective benefits of treatment choices. In this fashion, standardizing outcome measurement is a necessary step in transitioning to a value-based payment model.[13]

The transition to standardized outcome reporting already has occurred in other fields. The ICHOM has created standardized outcome measures for multiple other conditions, such as hip and knee osteoarthritis and congenital upper limb anomalies.[114,115] An international group of experts and patient representatives currently is developing a similar set of standardized outcomes for hand and wrist conditions.[116] There are several challenges to developing such an instrument, including the incorporation of subjective and objective patient-specific and injury-specific factors into a tool that is both responsive and translatable across countries and cultures. The recent transition to a patient-centered perspective and corresponding evolution of PROMs has been an important step in this process. CAT offers tremendous potential to efficiently apply instruments that are responsive yet concise.

The authors anticipate that the ICHOM Hand and Wrist Standard Set will guide DRF outcome measurement in the future and propose the following algorithm based on the currently available literature. These recommendations are summarized in **Table 3**. Pain should be measured independently using a VAS or NRS Scale. PROMs should be collected using one of the validated scoring systems. Performance measures, such as ROM and grip strength, and radiographic outcomes are important adjuncts that can offer objective data on residual disability and fracture healing. Complication reporting should be standardized and graded based on severity. Patient-specific and injury-specific factors that modify outcomes also should be accounted and adjusted for. Finally, a standardized timeline should be followed for measuring the aforementioned outcomes and electronic adjuncts should be used to decrease the burden to patients, providers, and researchers. Providing a comprehensive approach to DRF outcome measurement, the authors believe, can best determine optimal treatment algorithms in a value-based health care model.

CLINICS CARE POINTS

- Pain should be measured independently using a validated scale, such as the VAS, NRS, or PRWE subscale.
- PROMs should be collected using 1 of the validated scoring systems, such as the MHQ/bMHQ, DASH/QuickDASH, and PROMIS.
- Performance measures, such and ROM and grip strength, and radiographic outcomes are important adjuncts that can offer objective data on residual disability and fracture healing.
- Complication reporting should be standardized and graded based on severity.
- Patient-specific and injury-specific factors that modify outcomes should be adjusted for.

DISCLOSURE

The authors have nothing to disclose.

REFERENCES

1. Nellans KW, Kowalski E, Chung KC. The epidemiology of distal radius fractures. Hand Clin 2012; 28(2):113–25.
2. Shauver MJ, Yin H, Banerjee M, et al. Current and future national costs to medicare for the treatment of distal radius fracture in the elderly. J Hand Surg Am 2011;36(8):1282–7.
3. Chung KC, Spilson SV. The frequency and epidemiology of hand and forearm fractures in the United States. J Hand Surg Am 2001;26(5):908–15.
4. Waljee JF, Ladd A, Macdermid JC, et al. The hand surgery landscape a unified approach to outcomes assessment for distal radius fractures. J Hand Surg Am 2016;41(4):565–73.
5. Melton LJ, Amadio PC, Crowson CS, et al. Long-term trends in the incidence of distal forearm fractures. Osteoporos Int 1998;8(4):341–8.
6. Chung KC, Shauver MJ, Birkmeyer JD. Trends in the United States in the treatment of distal radial fractures in the elderly. J Bone Joint Surg Am 2009;91(8):1868–73.
7. Mellstrand-Navarro C, Pettersson HJ, Tornqvist H, et al. The operative treatment of fractures of the distal radius is increasing. Bone Joint J 2014;96-B(7):963–9.
8. Shauver MJ, Clapham PJ, Chung KC. An economic analysis of outcomes and complications of treating distal radius fractures in the elderly. J Hand Surg Am 2011;36(12). https://doi.org/10.1016/j.jhsa.2011.09.039.
9. Bonafede M, Espindle D, Bower AG. The direct and indirect costs of long bone fractures in a working age US population. J Med Econ 2013;16(1):169–78.
10. Porter ME. A strategy for health care reform–toward a value-based system. N Engl J Med 2009;361(2):109–12.
11. Porter ME. Value-based health care delivery. Ann Surg 2008;248(4):503–9.
12. Porter ME. What is value in health care? N Engl J Med 2010;363(26):2477–81.
13. Porter ME, Larsson S, Lee TH. Standardizing Patient Outcomes Measurement. N Engl J Med 2016;374(6):504–6.
14. Goldhahn J, Beaton D, Ladd A, et al. Recommendation for measuring clinical outcome in distal radius fractures: A core set of domains for standardized reporting in clinical practice and research. Arch Orthop Trauma Surg 2014;134(2):197–205.
15. Karantana A, Handoll HH, Sabouni A. Percutaneous pinning for treating distal radial fractures in adults. Cochrane Database Syst Rev 2020;2(2):CD006080.
16. Hoang-Kim A, Scott J, Micera G, et al. Functional assessment in patients with osteoporotic wrist fractures treated with external fixation: a review of randomized trials. Arch Orthop Trauma Surg 2009;129(1):105–11.
17. Diaz-Garcia RJ, Oda T, Shauver MJ, et al. A systematic review of outcomes and complications of treating unstable distal radius fractures in the elderly. J Hand Surg Am 2011;36(5):824–35.e2.
18. Chen Y, Chen X, Li Z, et al. Safety and Efficacy of Operative Versus Nonsurgical Management of Distal Radius Fractures in Elderly Patients: A Systematic Review and Meta-analysis. J Hand Surg Am 2016;41(3):404–13.
19. Chung KC, Shauver MJ. Measuring quality in health care and its implications for pay-for-performance initiatives. Hand Clin 2009;25(1):71–81, vii.
20. Gartland JJ, Werley CW. Evaluation of healed Colles' fractures. J Bone Joint Surg Am 1951;33A(4):895–907.
21. Sarmiento A, Pratt GW, Berry NC, et al. Colles' fractures. Functional bracing in supination. J Bone Joint Surg Am 1975;57(3):311–7. Available at: http://www.ncbi.nlm.nih.gov/pubmed/1123382. Accessed April 1, 2020.
22. Changulani M, Okonkwo U, Keswani T, et al. Outcome evaluation measures for wrist and hand - Which one to choose? Int Orthop 2008;32(1):1–6.
23. Green DP, O'Brien ET. Open reduction of carpal dislocations: indications and operative techniques. J Hand Surg Am 1978;3(3):250–65.

24. Cooney WP, Bussey R, Dobyns JH, et al. Difficult wrist fractures. Perilunate fracture-dislocations of the wrist. Clin Orthop Relat Res 1987;214:136–47.

25. Gupta S, Halai M, Al-Maiyah M, et al. Which measure should be used to assess the patient's functional outcome after distal radius fracture? Acta Orthop Belg 2014;80(1):116–8. Available at: http://www.ncbi.nlm.nih.gov/pubmed/24873095. Accessed March 30, 2020.

26. Amadio PC, Silverstein MD, Ilstrup DM, et al. Outcome after Colles fracture: the relative responsiveness of three questionnaires and physical examination measures. J Hand Surg Am 1996;21(5):781–7.

27. MacDermid JC, Richards RS, Donner A, et al. Responsiveness of the short form-36, disability of the arm, shoulder, and hand questionnaire, patient-rated wrist evaluation, and physical impairment measurements in evaluating recovery after a distal radius fracture. J Hand Surg Am 2000;25(2):330–40.

28. MacDermid JC, Turgeon T, Richards RS, et al. Patient Rating of Wrist Pain and Disability: A Reliable and Valid Measurement Tool. J Orthop Trauma 1998;12(8):577–86.

29. Mehta SP, MacDermid JC, Richardson J, et al. A systematic review of the measurement properties of the patient-rated wrist evaluation. J Orthop Sports Phys Ther 2015;45(4):289–98.

30. McKay SD, MacDermid JC, Roth JH, et al. Assessment of complications of distal radius fractures and development of a complication checklist. J Hand Surg Am 2001;26(5):916–22.

31. Curtin CM, Hernandez-Boussard T. Readmissions after treatment of distal radius fractures. J Hand Surg Am 2014;39(10):1926–32.

32. Mehta SP, Macdermid JC, Richardson J, et al. Baseline pain intensity is a predictor of chronic pain in individuals with distal radius fracture. J Orthop Sports Phys Ther 2015;45(2):119–27.

33. Amtmann D, Cook KF, Jensen MP, et al. Development of a PROMIS item bank to measure pain interference. Pain 2010;150(1):173–82.

34. Beaton DE, Wright JG, Katz JN, et al. Development of the QuickDASH: COmparison of three item-reduction approaches. J Bone Joint Surg Am 2005;87(5):1038–46.

35. Cook KF, Dunn W, Griffith JW, et al. Pain assessment using the NIH Toolbox. Neurology 2013;80(11 Suppl 3). https://doi.org/10.1212/wnl.0b013e3182872e80.

36. Hudak PL, Amadio PC, Bombardier C. Development of an upper extremity outcome measure: the DASH (disabilities of the arm, shoulder and hand) [corrected]. The Upper Extremity Collaborative Group (UECG). Am J Ind Med 1996;29(6):602–8.

37. Chung KC, Pillsbury MS, Walters MR, et al. Reliability and validity testing of the Michigan Hand Outcomes Questionnaire. J Hand Surg Am 1998;23(4):575–87.

38. MacDermid JC, Donner A, Richards RS, et al. Patient versus injury factors as predictors of pain and disability six months after a distal radius fracture. J Clin Epidemiol 2002;55(9):849–54.

39. Moore CM, Leonardi-Bee J. The prevalence of pain and disability one year post fracture of the distal radius in a UK population: a cross sectional survey. BMC Musculoskelet Disord 2008;9:129.

40. Kortlever JTP, Janssen SJ, van Berckel MMG, et al. What is the most useful questionnaire for measurement of coping strategies in response to nociception? Clin Orthop Relat Res 2015;473(11):3511–8.

41. MacDermid JC, Roth JH, McMurtry R. Predictors of time lost from work following a distal radius fracture. J Occup Rehabil 2007;17(1):47–62.

42. Bertakis KD, Azari R. Patient-centered care is associated with decreased health care utilization. J Am Board Fam Med 2011;24(3):229–39.

43. Schuind FA, Mouraux D, Robert C, et al. Functional and outcome evaluation of the hand and wrist. Hand Clin 2003;19(3):361–9.

44. MacDermid JC. Development of a scale for patient rating of wrist pain and disability. J Hand Ther 1996;9(2):178–83.

45. Kleinlugtenbelt YV, Krol RG, Bhandari M, et al. Are the patient-rated wrist evaluation (PRWE) and the disabilities of the arm, shoulder and hand (DASH) questionnaire used in distal radial fractures truly valid and reliable? Bone Joint Res 2018;7(1):36–45.

46. Redelmeier DA, Guyatt GH, Goldstein RS. Assessing the minimal important difference in symptoms: A comparison of two techniques. J Clin Epidemiol 1996;49(11):1215–9.

47. Walenkamp MMJ, de Muinck Keizer RJ, Goslings JC, et al. The Minimum Clinically Important Difference of the Patient-rated Wrist Evaluation Score for Patients With Distal Radius Fractures. Clin Orthop Relat Res 2015;473(10):3235–41.

48. Paranaíba VF, Dos Santos JBG, Raduan Neto J, et al. PRWE application in distal radius fracture: comparison and correlation with established outcomes. Rev Bras Ortop 2017;52(3):278–83.

49. Beaton DE, Katz JN, Fossel AH, et al. Measuring the whole or the parts? Validity, reliability, and responsiveness of the disabilities of the arm, shoulder and hand outcome measure in different regions of the upper extremity. J Hand Ther 2001;14(2):128–42.

50. Sorensen AA, Howard D, Tan WH, et al. Minimal clinically important differences of 3 patient-rated outcomes instruments. J Hand Surg Am 2013;38(4):641–9.

51. Franchignoni F, Vercelli S, Giordano A, et al. Minimal clinically important difference of the disabilities of the arm, shoulder and hand outcome measure (DASH) and its shortened version (quickDASH). J Orthop Sports Phys Ther 2014;44(1):30–9.

52. Smith-Forbes EV, Howell DM, Willoughby J, et al. Specificity of the minimal clinically important difference of the quick Disabilities of the Arm Shoulder and Hand (QDASH) for distal upper extremity conditions. J Hand Ther 2016;29(1):81–8 [quiz: 88].

53. Tyser AR, Beckmann J, Franklin JD, et al. Evaluation of the PROMIS physical function computer adaptive test in the upper extremity. J Hand Surg Am 2014;39(10):2047–51.e4.

54. Ware JE. Improvements in short-form measures of health status: introduction to a series. J Clin Epidemiol 2008;61(1):1–5.

55. Ware JE, Kosinski M, Keller SD. A 12-Item Short-Form Health Survey: Construction of Scales and Preliminary Tests of Reliability and Validity. Med Care 1996;34(3):220–33.

56. Halpern SD, Asch DA. Commentary: Improving response rates to mailed surveys: what do we learn from randomized controlled trials? Int J Epidemiol 2003;32(4):637–8.

57. Shauver MJ, Chung KC. The Michigan hand outcomes questionnaire after 15 years of field trial. Plast Reconstr Surg 2013;131(5):779e–87e.

58. Pap G, Angst F, Herren D, et al. Evaluation of wrist and hand handicap and postoperative outcome in rheumatoid arthritis. Hand Clin 2003;19(3):471–81.

59. Chung KC, Hamill JB, Walters MR, et al. The Michigan hand outcomes questionnaire (MHQ): Assessment of responsiveness to clinical change. Ann Plast Surg 1999;42(6):619–22.

60. Shauver MJ, Chung KC. The minimal clinically important difference of the Michigan hand outcomes questionnaire. J Hand Surg Am 2009;34(3):509–14.

61. London DA, Stepan JG, Calfee RP. Determining the michigan hand outcomes questionnaire minimal clinically important difference by means of three methods. Plast Reconstr Surg 2014;133(3):616–25.

62. Waljee JF, Kim HM, Burns PB, et al. Development of a brief, 12-item version of the Michigan Hand Questionnaire. Plast Reconstr Surg 2011;128(1):208–20.

63. Ware JE, Sherbourne CD. The MOS 36-item short-form health survey (Sf-36): I. conceptual framework and item selection. Med Care 1992;30(6):473–83.

64. Jenkinson C, Wright L, Coulter A. Criterion validity and reliability of the SF-36 in a population sample. Qual Life Res 1994;3(1):7–12.

65. Stucki G, Liang MH, Phillips C, et al. The Short Form-36 is preferable to the SIP as a generic health status measure in patients undergoing elective total hip arthroplasty. Arthritis Care Res 1995;8(3):174–81.

66. Anzarut A, Johnson JA, Rowe BH, et al. Radiologic and patient-reported functional outcomes in an elderly cohort with conservatively treated distal radius fractures. J Hand Surg Am 2004;29(6):1121–7.

67. Brogren E, Hofer M, Petranek M, et al. Relationship between distal radius fracture malunion and arm-related disability: a prospective population-based cohort study with 1-year follow-up. BMC Musculoskelet Disord 2011;12:9.

68. Jaremko JL, Lambert RGW, Rowe BH, et al. Do radiographic indices of distal radius fracture reduction predict outcomes in older adults receiving conservative treatment? Clin Radiol 2007;62(1):65–72.

69. Gandek B, Ware JE, Aaronson NK, et al. Cross-validation of item selection and scoring for the SF-12 Health Survey in nine countries: Results from the IQOLA Project. J Clin Epidemiol 1998;51(11):1171–8.

70. Cella D, Yount S, Rothrock N, et al. The Patient-Reported Outcomes Measurement Information System (PROMIS): progress of an NIH Roadmap cooperative group during its first two years. Med Care 2007;45(5 Suppl 1):S3–11.

71. Cella D, Riley W, Stone A, et al. The patient-reported outcomes measurement information system (PROMIS) developed and tested its first wave of adult self-reported health outcome item banks: 2005-2008. J Clin Epidemiol 2010;63(11):1179–94.

72. Overbeek CL, Nota SPFT, Jayakumar P, et al. The PROMIS physical function correlates with the QuickDASH in patients with upper extremity illness. Clin Orthop Relat Res 2015;473(1):311–7.

73. Cella D, Chang CH. A discussion of item response theory and its applications in health status assessment. Med Care 2000;38(9 Suppl):II66–72.

74. Cook KF, O'Malley KJ, Roddey TS. Dynamic assessment of health outcomes: Time to let the CAT out of the bag? Health Serv Res 2005;40(5 II):1694–711.

75. Rose M, Bjorner JB, Becker J, et al. Evaluation of a preliminary physical function item bank supported the expected advantages of the Patient-Reported Outcomes Measurement Information System (PROMIS). J Clin Epidemiol 2008;61(1):17–33.

76. Hung M, Stuart AR, Higgins TF, et al. Computerized Adaptive Testing Using the PROMIS Physical Function Item Bank Reduces Test Burden With Less Ceiling Effects Compared With the Short Musculoskeletal Function Assessment in Orthopaedic Trauma Patients. J Orthop Trauma 2014;28(8):439–43.

77. Hung M, Voss MW, Bounsanga J, et al. Examination of the PROMIS upper extremity item bank. J Hand Ther 2017;30(4):485–90.

78. Hung M, Clegg DO, Greene T, et al. Evaluation of the PROMIS physical function item bank in orthopaedic patients. J Orthop Res 2011;29(6):947–53.

79. Hays RD, Spritzer KL, Amtmann D, et al. Upper-extremity and mobility subdomains from the Patient-Reported Outcomes Measurement Information System (PROMIS) adult physical functioning item bank. Arch Phys Med Rehabil 2013;94(11):2291–6.

80. Beleckas CM, Padovano A, Guattery J, et al. Performance of Patient-Reported Outcomes Measurement Information System (PROMIS) Upper Extremity (UE) Versus Physical Function (PF) Computer Adaptive Tests (CATs) in Upper Extremity Clinics. J Hand Surg Am 2017;42(11):867–74.

81. Waljee JF, Carlozzi N, Franzblau LE, et al. Applying the patient-reported outcomes measurement information system to assess upper extremity function among children with congenital hand differences. Plast Reconstr Surg 2015;136(2):200e–7e.

82. Döring A-C, Nota SPFT, Hageman MGJS, et al. Measurement of upper extremity disability using the patient-reported outcomes measurement information system. J Hand Surg Am 2014;39(6):1160–5.

83. Sandvall B, Okoroafor UC, Gerull W, et al. Minimal Clinically Important Difference for PROMIS Physical Function in Patients With Distal Radius Fractures. J Hand Surg Am 2019;44(6):454–9.e1.

84. Hung M, Saltzman CL, Greene T, et al. The responsiveness of the PROMIS instruments and the qDASH in an upper extremity population. J Patient-reported Outcomes 2017;1(1):12.

85. Hall MJ, Ostergaard PJ, Dowlatshahi AS, et al. The Impact of Obesity and Smoking on Outcomes After Volar Plate Fixation of Distal Radius Fractures. J Hand Surg Am 2019;44(12):1037–49.

86. Haase SC, Chung KC. Management of malunions of the distal radius. Hand Clin 2012;28(2):207–16.

87. Kreder HJ, Hanel DP, McKee M, et al. X-ray film measurements for healed distal radius fractures. J Hand Surg Am 1996;21(1):31–9.

88. Friberg S, Lundström B. Radiographic measurements of the radio-carpal joint in normal adults. Acta Radiol Diagn (Stockh) 1976;17(2):249–56.

89. Graham TJ. Surgical correction of malunited fractures of the distal radius. J Am Acad Orthop Surg 1997;5(5):270–81.

90. Margaliot Z, Haase SC, Kotsis SV, et al. A meta-analysis of outcomes of external fixation versus plate osteosynthesis for unstable distal radius fractures. J Hand Surg Am 2005;30(6):1185–99.

91. Patel SP, Anthony SG, Zurakowski D, et al. Radiographic scoring system to evaluate union of distal radius fractures. J Hand Surg Am 2014;39(8):1471–9.

92. Young BT, Rayan GM. Outcome following nonoperative treatment of displaced distal radius fractures in low-demand patients older than 60 years. J Hand Surg Am 2000;25(1):19–28.

93. Ring D, Jupiter JB. Treatment of osteoporotic distal radius fractures. Osteoporos Int 2005;16(Suppl 2):S80–4.

94. Kasapinova K, Kamiloski V. Outcome evaluation in patients with distal radius fracture. Prilozi 2011;32(2):231–46.

95. Adams BD, Grosland NM, Murphy DM, et al. Impact of Impaired Wrist Motion on Hand and Upper-Extremity Performance. J Hand Surg Am 2003;28(6):898–903.

96. Bland MD, Beebe JA, Hardwick DD, et al. Restricted active range of motion at the elbow, forearm, wrist, or fingers decreases hand function. J Hand Ther 2008;21(3):268–74 [quiz: 275].

97. Chung KC, Haas A. Relationship between patient satisfaction and objective functional outcome after surgical treatment for distal radius fractures. J Hand Ther 2009;22(4):302–7 [quiz: 308].

98. Shauver MJ, Chang KW-C, Chung KC. Contribution of functional parameters to patient-rated outcomes after surgical treatment of distal radius fractures. J Hand Surg Am 2014;39(3):436–42.

99. Souer J-S, Lozano-Calderon SA, Ring D. Predictors of wrist function and health status after operative treatment of fractures of the distal radius. J Hand Surg Am 2008;33(2):157–63.

100. Becker SJE, Bruinsma WE, Guitton TG, et al. Interobserver Agreement of the Eaton-Glickel Classification for Trapeziometacarpal and Scaphotrapezial Arthrosis. J Hand Surg Am 2016;41(4):532–40.e1.

101. Lutz K, Yeoh KM, MacDermid JC, et al. Complications associated with operative versus nonsurgical treatment of distal radius fractures in patients aged 65 years and older. J Hand Surg Am 2014;39(7):1280–6.

102. Navarro CM, Pettersson HJ, Enocson A. Complications after distal radius fracture surgery: results from a Swedish nationwide registry study. J Orthop Trauma 2015;29(2):e36–42.

103. Griffin JW, Chhabra AB. Complications after volar plating of distal radius fractures. J Hand Surg Am 2014;39(6):1183–5 [quiz: 1186].

104. Mathews AL, Chung KC. Management of Complications of Distal Radius Fractures. Hand Clin 2015;31(2):205–15.

105. Walsh M, Davidovitch RI, Egol KA. Ethnic disparities in recovery following distal radial fracture. J Bone Joint Surg Am 2010;92(5):1082–7.

106. Paksima N, Pahk B, Romo S, et al. The association of education level on outcome after distal radius fracture. Hand (N Y) 2014;9(1):75–9.

107. Nelson GN, Stepan JG, Osei DA, et al. The impact of patient activity level on wrist disability after distal radius malunion in older adults. J Orthop Trauma 2015;29(4):195–200.

108. Soong M, van Leerdam R, Guitton TG, et al. Fracture of the distal radius: risk factors for complications after locked volar plate fixation. J Hand Surg Am 2011;36(1):3–9.

109. Chung KC, Kotsis SV, Kim HM. Predictors of functional outcomes after surgical treatment of distal radius fractures. J Hand Surg Am 2007;32(1):76–83.

110. Calfee RP, Shah CM, Canham CD, et al. The influence of insurance status on access to and utilization of a tertiary hand surgery referral center. J Bone Joint Surg Am 2012;94(23):2177–84.

111. Ostergaard PJ, Hall MJ, Rozental TD. Considerations in the Treatment of Osteoporotic Distal Radius Fractures in Elderly Patients. Curr Rev Musculoskelet Med 2019;12(1):50–6.

112. Dy CJ, Schmicker T, Tran Q, et al. The use of a tablet computer to complete the DASH questionnaire. J Hand Surg Am 2012;37(12):2589–94.

113. Yaffe M, Goyal N, Kokmeyer D, et al. The use of an iPad to collect patient-reported functional outcome measures in hand surgery. Hand 2015;10(3):522–8.

114. Rolfson O, Wissig S, van Maasakkers L, et al. Defining an International Standard Set of Outcome Measures for Patients With Hip or Knee Osteoarthritis: Consensus of the International Consortium for Health Outcomes Measurement Hip and Knee Osteoarthritis Working Group. Arthritis Care Res (Hoboken) 2016;68(11):1631–9.

115. ICHOM | Congenital Upper Limb Anomalies Standard Set. Available at: https://www.ichom.org/portfolio/congenital-upper-limb-anomalies/. Accessed March 30, 2020.

116. ICHOM | Hand & Wrist Conditions Standard Set | Measuring Outcomes. Available at: https://www.ichom.org/portfolio/hand-and-wrist-conditions/. Accessed March 30, 2020.

117. Sharpe F, Stevanovic M. Extra-articular distal radial fracture malunion. Hand Clin 2005;21(3):469–87.

What Is the Evidence in Treating Distal Radius Fractures in the Geriatric Population?

Lauren Fader, MD[a], Ethan Blackburn, MD[b],*

KEYWORDS

- Distal radius fracture • Geriatric • Elderly

KEY POINTS

- Distal radius fractures are common in the expanding geriatric population, making their treatment a matter of public health concern.
- When managing distal radius fractures in this population, it is important to differentiate between an active, chronologically older individual and a low-demand patient of a similar age, as treatment goals will differ.
- Quality of fracture reduction correlates with better function in young patients, but this does not necessarily apply in lower-demand elderly patients.
- Geriatric patients are a diverse population and must be managed on an individual basis with discussion of goals and expectations.

INTRODUCTION

Distal radius fractures are one of the most common injuries sustained by geriatric individuals. As the elderly population continues to grow, treating these injuries has become a matter of public health. Historically, these fractures were almost exclusively managed nonoperatively in a cast, but with the development of volar locked plating in the early 2000s, there has been a trend toward treating more geriatric distal radius fractures operatively.[1] Traditional conservative management is based on the assumption of low functional demands in elderly patients.[1] However, over the past few decades, the growing incidence of distal radius fractures has resulted from an elderly population increasing in numbers as well as activity level.[2]

Surgical and conservative treatment options have similar functional outcomes, yet the use of internal fixation, specifically volar locked plating, is increasing.[3-6] It has been hypothesized that this increase is due to multiple factors, including physician experience and preference, patient preferences, and evidence that volar locked plating provides enough stability for immediate range of motion while maintaining alignment and earlier use of the extremity.[1,7-9] This translates to faster recovery and return to independent living.

Ultimately, decision-making criteria for whether to treat an elderly patient surgically or conservatively is unclear. The most recent guidelines developed by the American Academy of Orthopedic Surgeons on distal radius fractures are inconclusive in their recommendation for or against surgical treatment of distal radius fractures in elderly patients.[10] Much of the existing data on this topic are obtained from studying younger patients. Some studies have focused on elderly patients,

[a] Department of Orthopaedic Surgery, University of Louisville, 550 South Jackson Street, ACB, 1st Floor, Louisville, KY 40202, USA; [b] Norton Healthcare, Hand and Upper Extremity Surgery, Louisville Arm and Hand, University of Louisville, Orthopaedic Surgery, 9880 Angies Way, Suite 350, Louisville, KY 40241, USA
* Corresponding author.
E-mail address: Ethan.blackburn@nortonhealthcare.org

Hand Clin 37 (2021) 229–237
https://doi.org/10.1016/j.hcl.2021.02.005
0749-0712/21/© 2021 Elsevier Inc. All rights reserved.

but most included lower-demand, medically complicated patients.[4,11,12] Fewer data exist on geriatric patients who are active and higher demand.

EPIDEMIOLOGY

Distal radius fractures account for up to 18% of all fractures in patients older than 65, with only hip fractures occurring more frequently in this age group.[1,13,14] Many factors contribute to this high rate, including changes in bone structure, increased activity levels, and metabolic bone disease.[2]

Low-energy trauma is the most common cause of fractures in the elderly, specifically falls from a standing height onto an outstretched hand. Many distal radius fractures occur when an individual attempts to break a fall by putting out the hands. It has been suggested that these injuries may occur more frequently in those who are cognitively and neuromuscularly intact, rather than those with dementia. These individuals have the awareness to try to stop a fall, rather than falling on the side of their arm or leg, which would lead to a proximal humerus or hip fracture.[15,16]

Women have a higher risk of distal radius fractures than men in the geriatric population. Brogren and colleagues[17] found that elderly women had almost 5 times more distal radius fractures than elderly men. They also found that the distal radius fracture incidence for women increased rapidly from 50 years of age and older, almost doubling every 10 years until 90 years of age.

With the increasing incidence of distal radius fractures in the geriatric population comes a surge in short- and long-term costs for managing these injuries. Shauver and colleagues[13] analyzed these costs specific to the elderly community and found that in 2007, Medicare paid $170 million in distal radius fracture–related payments. They projected that total direct payments could reach $240 million if the utilization of internal fixation in treating distal radius fractures continues to increase. This value does not include secondary costs such as medications, loss of time at work, and loss of independence.

CONSIDERATIONS IN ELDERLY PATIENTS

One of the most difficult aspects of managing geriatric patients with a distal radius fracture is reconciling the disconnect between physiologic and chronologic age of the patient. How should we define "geriatric," "elderly," or "low demand"? There is no numeric value assigned to these terms, and 2 patients of the same age can differ significantly in terms of health status and functional demands. Elderly individuals today are more active than ever.[1] It is increasingly difficult to differentiate between the active, chronologically older individual who will place high demands on a recovering injured wrist, and the low-demand patient of a similar age who may be satisfied without anatomic restoration of the fractured wrist.[2] In the current literature, patients are rarely stratified based on infirmity and activity level.[18] Patients older than 70 can be very different from those between 60 and 70 years old, yet both groups may be considered "elderly."[19]

A close correlation between restoration of anatomy and functional outcome has been shown to exist in younger patients.[20,21] At long-term follow-up of 12 to 14 years, Ali and colleagues[22] found that adults 18 to 65 years of age with malunion of a distal radial fracture had greater activity limitations, worse pain, and lower satisfaction than those who healed without malunion. Conversely, studies focused on geriatric patients suggested that they can be treated conservatively, even with an unstable fracture pattern, because there is less connection between fracture reduction and functional outcome compared with younger cohorts.[11,12,23] It is generally accepted that open reduction internal fixation (ORIF) provides more stable fixation and facilitates earlier range of motion than nonoperative treatment, but the clinical significance of this has not been proven.[24]

Osteoporosis affects severity and complication rates related to distal radius fractures in the elderly. A distal radius fracture sustained during a fall from standing height onto an outstretched hand is considered a "fragility fracture" and diagnostic of osteoporosis. A study by Clayton and colleagues[25] found that decreased bone mineral density was associated with more severe intra-articular fractures. It has also been shown that patients with osteoporosis are at increased risk of early instability, malunion, and late carpal malalignment following distal radius fracture compared with patients with normal bone mineral density.[25,26]

MANAGEMENT

For patients older than 50, important factors to consider when deciding on a management strategy include fracture pattern, age, daily activity level and lifestyle requirements, hand dominance, presence of osteoporosis, and current medical conditions.[16,27] In addition, questions for patients and providers when considering a certain treatment relate to the long-term benefit on function, mortality, and the risk of complications.[28]

Physician preferences and experience affect management as well. For example, patients evaluated by members of the American Society for Surgery of the Hand or surgeons less than 10 years out of residency are more likely to have ORIF.[29] Patient preference plays a role in management as well. In the Wrist and Radius Injury Surgical Trial (WRIST), a multicenter, international, randomized controlled trial of treatment for displaced extra-articular and intra-articular distal radius fractures in patients 60 years and older, 60% of eligible patients study-wide refused to enroll, with the most common reason for refusal being preference for a specific treatment.[7]

Nevertheless, treatment decisions are rarely made by the surgeon or patient alone. It is typically a cooperative process.[7] In all cases, regardless of age, the surgeon and patient should have the overall goals of treatment in mind: a painless extremity with good function, and acceptable risk for potential complications.

Nonsurgical

Specific protocols for nonoperative management of distal radius fractures vary somewhat depending on provider preferences, but in general, the same principles are followed. Minimally displaced fractures can be initially placed directly into a short arm splint. If the fracture is significantly displaced, closed reduction is performed under some form of anesthesia before placement in a sugar tong splint. A splint that includes the elbow limits protonation and supination. It is important to leave the metacarpophalangeal joints free to allow for finger range of motion. Careful attention should be given to the fragile skin of elderly patients during reduction and splinting, as skin can tear easily.

The patient is transitioned from the splint to a short arm cast in the first 1 to 2 weeks and should be assessed with radiographs weekly for the first several weeks. Patients require close follow-up to monitor for collapse and secondary displacement. A study by Beumer and McQueen[30] found that 53 of 60 distal radius fractures in patients who were elderly, low-demand, or had dementia who were initially closed reduced went on to malunion. Patients should be counseled on the risks of displacement and possible cosmetic deformity.

Identifying factors that place patients at a higher risk for secondary displacement is important when recommending a course of treatment. In 1989, Lafontaine and colleagues[31] named 5 factors predictive of fracture instability: dorsal comminution, intra-articular extension, initial dorsal angulation greater than 20°, an associated ulna fracture, and age older than 60 years. The investigators stated that a fracture is at risk for secondary displacement if 3 or more factors are present. The factors identified by Lafontaine remain popular as predictors of instability, but a recent meta-analysis demonstrated that associated ulna fractures, dorsal angulation greater than 20°, and intra-articular fractures do not have an increased risk of secondary displacement. These investigators found age older than 60 to 65 years, female gender, and dorsal comminution to be significant predictors of secondary displacement.[32]

Jung and colleagues[33] analyzed a cohort of patients with distal radius fractures treated conservatively to provide prognostic factors for loss of initial closed reduction. They specifically looked at 3 of the "most controversial" risk factors: age, dorsal comminution, and degree of initial displacement. They concluded that degree of initial displacement is the most important predictive factor for secondary displacement and suggested that older patients are at high risk for late secondary displacement. This supports the findings of Makhni and colleagues,[34] who reported that increases in age significantly increase the rate of redisplacement in fractures that were subject to initial closed reduction ($P = .03$).

Distal radius fractures can collapse and develop a malunion when treated conservatively, especially those with the risk factors described previously, but multiple studies have demonstrated that many elderly patients still have adequate function despite the development of a malunion.[1,11,12,35]

Surgical

Operative treatment options for distal radius fractures in elderly patients include closed or open reduction with fixation by various methods such as external fixator, percutaneous pinning with K-wires, volar or dorsal locking plate, or dorsal bridge plate. Combinations of plating and percutaneous or external fixation can also be used if necessary.

Fragment-specific fixation is occasionally indicated, especially in cases with volar lunate facet fractures, which can be difficult to capture with standard volar locking plates. Failure to stabilize this fragment leads to volar subluxation of the fragment and the carpus. Dorsal bridge plating is a useful technique in certain scenarios, such as fractures in polytrauma patients who require more urgent stabilization due to other injuries, fractures extending into the diaphysis, and comminuted fractures in osteoporotic patients.[16] The dorsal bridge plate allows patients to use the injured upper extremity to assist with mobilization.

The addition of bone graft may be beneficial in some elderly patients with osteoporotic bone, comminuted fractures, and/or metaphyseal bone loss to provide additional structural stability. Ozer and Chung[36] summarize the use of bone grafts or substitutes in distal radius fractures. They emphasize that bone quality, size of the bone defect, blood supply to the fracture site, and method of immobilization all affect the healing process and maintenance of reduction in distal radius fractures. They recommend iliac crest bone graft in cases of significant bone loss or nonunion, and calcium phosphate and allograft bone chips in all other cases.[36]

OUTCOMES

High-quality studies looking to identify conditions that will guide decision-making in treating distal radius fractures in active elderly patients are difficult. Numerous factors influence treatment strategies and affect outcomes. In addition, long-term follow-up is needed to truly evaluate the development of negative sequelae, such as radiocarpal and midcarpal arthritis or dorsal intercalated segment instability, among others.

Clinically, the most desirable result of treatment is a pain-free wrist with good function. Pain and function are measured in existing literature using visual analogue pain scale and/or functional assessment tools such as the Disabilities of the Arm, Shoulder, and Hand (DASH) score, the Patient-Rated Wrist Evaluation (PRWE) score, the Green and O'Brien score, and the Michigan Hand Outcomes Questionnaire. Other outcomes frequently investigated include radiographic parameters (radial tilt, radial inclination, radial height, and articular step-off), grip strength, and range of motion. These objective radiographic variables, however, do not always correlate with pain and function.[37] There is general consensus that quality of reduction correlates with function in young patients, but this does not always apply in the lower-demand, geriatric population.

EVIDENCE

In 2009, Arora and colleagues[27] retrospectively examined 114 unstable dorsally displaced distal radius fractures in patients older than 70 years. Of note, they only included patients who were independent and able to attend follow-up visits on their own. This likely introduced some bias toward higher-demand geriatric patients. Fractures were considered unstable if they lost reduction during the first 2 weeks after initial reduction and immobilization. ORIF with volar plate fixation was recommended to all patients, but 61 declined and were treated with plaster cast immobilization. The mean follow-up time for the operative group was 51 months and 62 months for the cast group. At final follow-up, there were no differences in active motion, grip strength, DASH score, PRWE score, or Green and O'Brien score between the 2 groups. Patients in the cast group had more radiographic evidence of radiocarpal arthritis, but less pain. Thirteen percent of patients in the operative group developed a complication, with 11% requiring secondary surgical procedures. Eight percent of patients in the cast group developed complex regional pain syndrome. This was the only type of complication identified in this group. Of the cast patients, 77% were noted to have a prominent ulnar head at final follow-up, but no patient was unhappy with their wrist appearance.

Two years later, the same group published a prospective, randomized trial comparing nonoperative treatment with volar locked plating for distal radius fractures in 73 patients older than 65.[4] Again, they only included patients who were living independently, excluding low-functioning individuals. All patients had at least 12 months of clinical and radiographic follow-up. There were no significant differences in range of motion or pain level between the 2 groups through the entire follow-up period. Patients in the operative group had lower DASH and PRWE scores initially, indicating better wrist function, but there were no differences at 6 and 12 months. Grip strength was better in the operative group at all time points. Complications were more frequent in the operative group (36% vs 14%). Seventy-eight percent of patients in the cast group had a prominent ulnar head, but no patient was dissatisfied with the appearance of the wrist.

A retrospective study from Turkey reviewed 49 patients older than 60 with complex intra-articular (AO type C) distal radius fractures who were treated with either volar locked plating or cast immobilization.[6] Patients were followed for at least 12 months. The operative group had better grip strength and radiographic parameters at the end of follow-up, but there was no significant difference in quick DASH score or range of motion between the 2 groups.

In 2018, Martinez-Mendez and colleagues[19] published a randomized prospective study comparing casting versus volar locked plating for intra-articular distal radius fractures in patients older than 60. Patients were followed for at least 24 months. At final follow-up, the operative group had better PRWE and DASH scores compared with the casting group. There was no difference in wrist flexion and extension or grip strength, but protonation and supination were significantly greater in the surgical group ($P = .01$). All radiological parameters were better overall in the surgical group. The only parameter to not reach statistical significance was volar tilt ($P = .08$). More patients in the casting group than the surgical group had articular step-off >2 mm (26% vs 8%), but there was no association between articular incongruity and PRWE score. There was no significant difference in observed radiocarpal degenerative changes between the 2 groups at final follow-up. The investigators concluded that functional outcomes and quality of life were better after volar plating compared with conservative treatment, due in large part to restoration of the articular surface and recovery of radial inclination and ulnar variance.

A prospective cohort study of nonfrail elderly patients with distal radius fractures looked to determine the influence of treatment and radiographic parameters on patient-reported functional outcomes.[38] This study by Larouche and colleagues[38] was unique in that patients older than 55 years were stratified based on a clinical frailty scale to specifically investigate those patients who are chronologically older but may be physiologically "young." Patients were treated with closed reduction and casting or ORIF as per the treating surgeons' decision. Radiographic parameters as well as DASH, Short Form 36, and PRWE scores were recorded at baseline and through follow-up. They found no difference in outcomes based on treatment choice between casting and ORIF. They did find that persistent ulnar positivity and the presence of an articular step or gap greater than 2 mm on final radiographs were associated with worse functional outcome.

COMPLICATIONS

Complication rates published in the literature range widely from 0% to 47%, and methods for reporting complications are not consistent.[4,39,40] Complications can occur with any treatment modality, and they affect not only outcomes and quality of life, but also increase costs to the health care system. The most common complications associated with distal radius fractures include median nerve neuropathy, complex regional pain syndrome, tendon rupture, and malunion. These complications may or may not require secondary surgery.

Much of these data come from studies comparing different treatments, and reporting complications is a secondary aim. McKay and colleagues[41] developed a checklist for standardizing data collection, which includes a classification

system for all complications and allows for the assessment of complication severity. The goal of the checklist is to examine distal radius fracture complications in a systematic way.

Lutz and colleagues[39] looked to compare complication rates for distal radius fractures treated operatively versus nonoperatively in patients older than 65 years using the checklist developed by McKay and colleagues.[41] The most common complication overall was median nerve neuropathy (8% of all patients), followed by surgical site infection and complex regional pain syndrome. They found a higher rate of complications in patients treated operatively compared with nonoperatively (29% vs 17%). In the operative group, pin track infections in patients treated with external fixation was the most common complication. There was a significantly greater number of malunions in the nonoperative group ($P = <0.001$). A subset of patients had 1-year follow-up PRWE scores, and in those patients, there was no significant difference in patient-reported pain and disability between the 2 groups.

Chung and colleagues[40] also attempted to characterize complications following treatment of distal radius fractures in older patients through a secondary analysis of the WRIST. Complications included nerve complications, bone and/or joint complications, and tendon complications. All were classified as mild, moderate, or severe per the checklist developed by McKay and colleagues.[41] Other measures included comorbidities, preinjury functional status, malunion, delayed union, and arthritis. At final analysis, 287 patients were available with complication data. The rates of any type of complication were lowest in the volar locking plate group. The casting group had higher rates of any complication, likely from a higher rate of malunions. Most complications happened early in the follow-up period. Of the 3 surgical groups (volar locked plating, percutaneous pinning, or bridging external fixation), external fixation had the highest complication rates. The investigators concluded that external fixation has more moderate complications than volar locked plating, and pinning has higher rates of infection. They concluded that in all cases, choice of treatment in older patients should be specific to individual goals and balance functional outcomes and complication risks.

A systematic review by Diaz-Garcia and colleagues[42] looked at outcomes and complications in treating distal radius fractures in elderly individuals. They compared complications among 5 common techniques for treating these injuries: volar locked plating, nonbridging external fixation, bridging external fixation, percutaneous pinning, and cast immobilization. They found bridging external fixation to have the highest rates of minor and major complications not requiring surgery. Volar locked plating had the highest rate of major complications requiring surgery. Cast immobilization had the fewest complications in all categories.

DISCUSSION

Distal radius fractures in elderly individuals are a major public health issue because of the high prevalence in this population, the great cost associated with their care, and the resultant temporary or permanent loss of independence.[43] Multiple studies have demonstrated that operative treatment often results in better radiographic parameters and grip strength, but there seems to be no difference in clinical and functional outcomes.[3,4,6,27,44] On the other hand, there are also studies suggesting that operative treatment results in superior outcomes and fewer complications.[19,45]

Clearly, there are still questions regarding how to best manage these patients to minimize loss of function and complications. The WRIST study group was formed in 2009 with the goal of answering some of these difficult treatment questions. As referenced previously, WRIST is a randomized clinical trial of treatment for displaced extra-articular and intra-articular distal radius fractures in patients 60 years and older. Patients in the trial were enrolled at 24 sites in the United States, Canada, and Singapore from 2012 through 2016. Participants with fractures requiring surgical fixation who were enrolled in the study either opted for surgical treatment or elected for nonoperative treatment with casting. The surgical patients were randomized to receive 1 of 3 treatments: volar locked plating, percutaneous pinning, or external fixation with or without supplemental pinning. The multicenter clinical trial has a rigorous study protocol with a diverse patient sample and a large number of patients to detect smaller treatment effects.[2] This type of large-scale, multicenter trial with long-term follow-up is necessary to improve treatment strategies and develop preventive measures that target this serious injury.

Future studies need to have long-term follow-up to be able to assess the prevalence, natural history, and symptoms of posttraumatic arthritis in elderly individuals and the influence of operative treatment. Furthermore, healthy, active patients should be analyzed separately from frail or low-demand individuals.[18] Finally, it would be beneficial to more clearly define objective factors to help surgeons determine who is low demand or frail versus those whose functional demand is higher despite advanced age. Efforts to

standardize this definition may assist in designing future studies.

SUMMARY

In the literature, there is no consensus on how to choose between surgical and conservative management of distal radius fractures in the geriatric population. We know radiographic outcomes are improved with volar locked plating, but this does not necessarily translate to long-term functional outcomes in elderly patients.

Geriatric patients are a diverse population with respect to functional demands, independence, bone quality, and coexisting medical conditions. One treatment does not fit all, and these patients must be managed on an individualized basis. Discussing goals and expectations with the patient can allow for a cooperative decision-making process to determine the best course for each individual.

CLINICS CARE POINTS

- Distal radius fractures are the second most common fracture sustained by patients older than 65, after hip fractures. As the elderly population continues to grow, treating these injuries is a matter of public health.

- Elderly patients today are more active than ever. When managing distal radius fractures in this population, it is important to differentiate between an active, chronologically older individual and a low-demand patient of a similar age, as treatment goals will differ.

- Since the development of volar locked plating in the early 2000s, more geriatric distal radius fractures are treated operatively. Clear evidence that this treatment modality is superior to nonoperative treatment has yet to be delivered.

- There is general consensus that quality of fracture reduction correlates with better function in young patients, but this does not necessarily apply in lower-demand elderly patients.

- Large-scale, multicenter trials, such as the WRIST, with long-term follow-up are necessary to improve prevention strategies and guide treatment of distal radius fractures in geriatric patients.

- Defining objective factors to help surgeons determine which patients are frail or low demand versus those with higher functional demands despite advanced age will assist in treating patients as well as designing future studies.

- Geriatric patients are a diverse population and must be managed on an individual basis. Open discussion between provider and patient or caregiver regarding goals and expectations allows for cooperative decision-making to formulate the best course for each individual.

ACKNOWLEDGMENTS

The WRIST group consists of the following: *Michigan Medicine (Coordinating Center):* Kevin C. Chung, MD, MS (Principal Investigator); H. Myra Kim, ScD (Study Biostatistician); Steven C. Haase, MD; Jeffrey N. Lawton, MD; John R. Lien, MD; Adeyiza O. Momoh, MD; Kagan Ozer, MD; Erika D. Sears, MD, MS; Jennifer F. Waljee, MD, MPH; Matthew S. Brown, MD (now at Basin Orthopedic Surgery Specialists); Hoyune E. Cho, MD; Brett F. Michelotti, MD (now at University of Wisconsin Health); Sunitha Malay, MPH (Study Coordinator); Melissa J. Shauver, MPH (Study Coordinator). *Beth Israel Deaconess Medical Center:* Tamara D. Rozental, MD (Co-Investigator); Paul T. Appleton, MD; Edward K. Rodriguez, MD, PhD; Laura N. Deschamps, DO; Lindsay Mattfolk, BA; Katiri Wagner. *Brigham and Women's Hospital*: Philip Blazar, MD (Co-Investigator); Brandon E. Earp, MD; W. Emerson Floyd; Dexter L. Louie, BS. *Duke Health:* Fraser J. Leversedge, MD (Co-Investigator); Marc J. Richard, MD; David, S. Ruch, MD; Suzanne Finley, CRC; Cameron Howe, CRC; Maria Manson; Janna Whitfield, BS. *Fraser Health Authority:* Bertrand H. Perey, MD (Co-Investigator); Kelly Apostle, MD, FRCSC; Dory Boyer, MD, FRCSC; Farhad Moola, MD, FRCSC; Trevor Stone, MD, FRCSC; Darius Viskontas, MD, FRCSC; Mauri Zomar, CCRP; Karyn Moon; Raely Pritchard. *HealthPartners Institute for Education and Research:* Loree K. Kalliainen, MD, MA (Co-Investigator, now at University of North Carolina Health Care); Christina M. Ward, MD (Co-Investigator); James W. Fletcher, MD; Cherrie A. Heinrich, MD; Katharine S. Pico, MD; Ashish Y. Mahajan, MD; Brian W. Hill, MD; Sandy Vang, BA. *Johns Hopkins Medicine:* Dawn M. Laporte, MD (Co-Investigator); Erik A. Hasenboehler, MD; Scott D. Lifchez, MD; Greg M. Osgood, MD; Babar Shafiq, MD, MS; Jaimie T. Shores, MD; Vaishali Laljani. *Kettering Health Network:* H. Brent Bamberger, DO (Co-Investigator); Timothy W. Harman, DO; David W. Martineau, MD; Carla Robinson, PA-C, MPAS; Brandi Palmer, MS, PC, CCRP. *London Health Sciences Center:* Ruby Grewal, MD, MS (Co-Investigator); Ken A. Faber, MD; Joy C. MacDermid, PhD (Study Epidemiologist); Kate Kelly, MSc, MPH; Katrina Munro; Joshua I. Vincent, PT, PhD. *Massachusetts General Hospital:* David Ring, MD, PhD (Co-Investigator, now at University of Texas Health Austin); Jesse B. Jupiter, MD, MA; Abigail Finger, BA; Jillian S. Gruber, MD; Rajesh K. Reddy, BA; Taylor M. Pong; Emily R. Thornton, BSc. *Mayo Clinic:* David G. Dennison, MD (Co-Investigator); Sanjeev Kakar, MD; Marco Rizzo, MD; Alexander Y. Shin, MD; Tyson L. Scrabeck, CCRP. *The MetroHealth System:* Kyle Chepla, MD (Co-Investigator); Kevin Malone, MD; Harry A. Hoyen, MD; Blaine Todd Bafus, MD; Roderick B. Jordan, MD; Bram Kaufman, MD; Ali Totonchil, MD; Dana R. Hromyak, BS, RRT; Lisa Humbert, RN. *National University of Singapore*: Sandeep Sebastin, MCh (Co-Investigator), Sally Tay. *Northwell Health*: Kate W. Nellans, MD, MPH (Co-Investigator); Sara L. Merwin, MPH. *Norton Healthcare:* Ethan W. Blackburn, MD (Co-Investigator); Sandra J. Hanlin, APRN, NP-C; Barbara Patterson, BSN, CCRC. *OrthoCarolina Research Institute:* R. Glenn Gaston, MD (Co-Investigator); R. Christopher Cadderdon, MD; Erika Gordon Gantt, MD; John S. Gaul, MD; Daniel R. Lewis, MD; Bryan J. Loeffler, MD; Lois K. Osier, MD; Paul C. Perlik, MD; W. Alan Ward, MD; Benjamin Connell, BA, CCRC; Pricilla Haug, BA, CCRC; Caleb Michalek, BS, CCRC. *Pan Am Clinic/University of Manitoba:* Tod A. Clark, MD, MSc, FRCSC(Co-Investigator); Sheila McRae, MSc, PhD. *University of Connecticut Health:* Jennifer Moriatis Wolf, MD (Co-Investigator, now at University of Chicago Medicine); Craig M. Rodner, MD; Katy Coyle, RN. *University of Oklahoma Medicine:* Thomas P. Lehman, MD, PT (Co-Investigator); Yuri C. Lansinger, MD; Gavin D. O'Mahony, MD; Kathy Carl, BA, CCRP; Janet Wells. *University of Pennsylvania Health System:* David J. Bozentka, MD (Co-Investigator); L. Scott Levin, MD; David P. Steinberg, MD; Annamarie D. Horan, PhD; Denise Knox, BS; Kara Napolitano, BS. *University of Pittsburgh Medical Center:* John Fowler, MD (Co-Investigator); Robert Goitz, MD; Cathy A. Naccarelli; Joelle Tighe. *University of Rochester:* Warren C. Hammert, MD, DDS (Co-Investigator); Allison W. McIntyre, MPH; Krista L. Noble; Kaili Waldrick. *University of Washington Medicine:* Jeffery B. Friedrich, MD (Co-Investigator); David Bowman; Angela Wilson. *Wake Forest Baptist Health:* Zhongyu Li, MD, PhD (Co-Investigator); L. Andrew Koman, MD; Benjamin R. Graves, MD; Beth P. Smith, PhD; Debra Bullard.

DISCLOSURES

The authors have no commercial or financial conflicts of interest. No funding was received for this project.

REFERENCES

1. Chung KC, Shauver MJ, Birkmeyer JD. Trends in the United States in the treatment of distal radial fractures in the elderly. J Bone Joint Surg Am 2009. https://doi.org/10.2106/JBJS.H.01297.

2. Nellans KW, Kowalski E, Chung KC. The epidemiology of distal radius fractures. Hand Clin 2012; 28(2):113–25.

3. Egol KA, Walsh M, Romo-Cardoso S, et al. Distal radial fractures in the elderly: operative compared with nonoperative treatment. J Bone Joint Surg Am 2010;92(9):1851–7.

4. Arora R, Lutz M, Deml C, et al. A prospective randomized trial comparing nonoperative treatment with volar locking plate fixation for displaced and unstable distal radial fractures in patients sixty-five years of age and older. Orthopedics 2012;35(1):50–1.

5. Chen Y, Chen X, Li Z, et al. Safety and efficacy of operative versus nonsurgical management of distal radius fractures in elderly patients: a systematic review and meta-analysis. J Hand Surg Am 2016; 41(3):404–13.

6. Zengin EC, Ozcan C, Aslan C, et al. Cast immobilization versus volar locking plate fixation of AO type C distal radial fractures in patients aged 60 years and older. Acta Orthop Traumatol Turc 2019; 53(1):15–8.

7. Nasser JS, Huetteman HE, Shauver MJ, et al. Older patient preferences for internal fixation after a distal radius fracture: a qualitative study from the wrist and radial injury surgical trial (WRIST). Plast Reconstr Surg 2018. https://doi.org/10.1097/PRS.0000000000004454.

8. Shauver MJ, Clapham PJ, Chung KC, et al. An economic analysis of outcomes and complications of treating distal radius fractures in the elderly. J Hand Surg 2011;36:1912–8.

9. Rozental TD, Blazar PE, Franko OI, et al. Functional outcomes for unstable distal radial fractures treated with open reduction and internal fixation or closed reduction and percutaneous fixation: a prospective randomized trial. J Bone Joint Surg Am 2009;91(8): 1837–46.

10. Murray J, Gross L. Treatment of distal radius fractures. J Am Acad Orthop Surg 2013;21(8):502–5.

11. Anzarut A, Johnson JA, Rowe BH, et al. Radiologic and patient-reported functional outcomes in an elderly cohort with conservatively treated distal radius fractures. J Hand Surg 2004;1121. https://doi.org/10.1016/j.jhsa.2004.07.002.

12. Young BT. Outcome following nonoperative treatment of displaced distal radius fractures in low-demand patients older than 60 years. J Hand Surg Am 2000;25(1):19–28.

13. Shauver MJ, Yin H, Banerjee M, et al. Current and future national costs to medicare for the treatment of distal radius fracture in the elderly. J Hand Surg 2011;36:1282–7.

14. Chung KC, Shauver MJ, Yin H, et al. Variations in the use of internal fixation for distal radial fracture in the united states medicare population. J Bone Joint Surg Am 2011. https://doi.org/10.2106/JBJS.J.012802.

15. Degoede KM, Ashton-Miller JA, Schultz AB. Fall-related upper body injuries in the older adult: a review of the biomechanical issues. J Biomech 2003; 36:1043–53.

16. Levin LS, Rozell JC, Pulos N. Distal radius fractures in the elderly. J Am Acad Orthop Surg 2017;25(3): 179–87.

17. Brogren E, Petranek M, Atroshi I. Incidence and characteristics of distal radius fractures in a southern Swedish region. BMC Musculoskelet Disord 2007. https://doi.org/10.1186/1471-2474-8-48.

18. Brogan DM, Ruch DS. Distal radius fractures in the elderly. J Hand Surg Am 2015;40(6):1217–9.

19. Martinez-Mendez D, Lizaur-Utrilla A, de-Juan-Herrero J. Intra-articular distal radius fractures in elderly patients: a randomized prospective study of casting versus volar plating. J Hand Surg Eur 2018;43(2):142–7.

20. Kopylov P, Johnell O, Redlund-johnell I, et al. Fractures of the distal end of the radius in young adults: a 30-year follow-up. J Hand Surg Am 1993;18(1):45–9.

21. Knirk JL, D4 M, Jupiter JB. Intra-articular fractures of the distal end of the radius in young adults. J Bone Joint Surg Am 1986;68(5):791.

22. Ali M, Brogren E, Wagner P, et al. Association between distal radial fracture malunion and patient-reported activity limitations. J Bone Joint Surg Am 2018;100-A(8):633–9.

23. Hohmann E, Meta M, Navalgund V, et al. The relationship between radiological alignment of united distal radius fractures and functional and patient-perceived outcomes in elderly patients. J Orthop Surg 2017;25(1):1–6.

24. Mauck BM, Swigler CW. Evidence-based review of distal radius fractures. Orthop Clin North Am 2018. https://doi.org/10.1016/j.ocl.2017.12.001.

25. Clayton RAE, Gaston MS, Ralston SH, et al. Association between decreased bone mineral density and severity of distal radial fractures. J Bone Joint Surg Am 2009;91(3):613–9.

26. Fitzpatrick SK, Casemyr NE, Zurakowski D, et al. The effect of osteoporosis on outcomes of operatively treated distal radius fractures. J Hand Surg 2012;37:2027–34.

27. Arora R, Gabl M, Gschwentner M, et al. A comparative study of clinical and radiologic outcomes of unstable Colles type distal radius fractures in patients older than 70 years: Nonoperative treatment versus volar locking plating. J Orthop Trauma 2009;23(4):237–42.

28. Vannabouathong C, Hussain N, Guerra-Farfan E, et al. Interventions for distal radius fractures: a network meta-analysis of randomized trials. J Am Acad Orthop Surg 2019;27(13):E596–605.

29. Wrist and Radius Injury Surgical Trial (WRIST) Study Group. Reflections 1 year into the 21-Center National Institutes of Health–funded WRIST study: a primer on conducting a multicenter clinical trial. J Hand Surg Am 2013;38(6):1194–201.

30. Beumer A, McQueen MM. Fractures of the distal radius in low-demand elderly patients: closed reduction of no value in 53 of 60 wrists. Acta Orthop Scand 2003;74(1):98–100.

31. Lafontaine M, Hardy D, Delince P. Stability assessment of distal radius fractures. Injury 1989;20(4):208–10.

32. Walenkamp MMJ, Aydin S, Mulders MAM, et al. Predictors of unstable distal radius fractures: a systematic review and meta-analysis. J Hand Surg Eur 2014;41(5):501–15.

33. Jung H-W, Hong H, Jung HJ, et al. Redisplacement of distal radius fracture after initial closed reduction: analysis of prognostic factors. Clin Orthop Surg 2015;7(3):377–82.

34. Makhni EC, Ewald TJ, Kelly S, et al. Effect of patient age on the radiographic outcomes of distal radius fractures subject to nonoperative treatment. J Hand Surg Am 2008. https://doi.org/10.1016/j.jhsa.2008.04.031.

35. Grewal R, Macdermid JC. The risk of adverse outcomes in extra-articular distal radius fractures is increased with malalignment in patients of all ages but mitigated in older patients. 2007. Available at: www.eradius.com. Accessed December 27, 2019.

36. Ozer K, Chung KC. The use of bone grafts and substitutes in the treatment of distal radius fractures. Hand Clin 2012. https://doi.org/10.1016/j.hcl.2012.02.004.

37. Kwok IHY, Leung F, Yuen G. Assessing results after distal radius fracture treatment: a comparison of objective and subjective tools. Geriatr Orthop Surg Rehabil 2011. https://doi.org/10.1177/2151458511422701.

38. Larouche J, Pike J, Slobogean GP, et al. Determinants of functional outcome in distal radius fractures in high-functioning patients older than 55 years. J Orthop Trauma 2016;30(8):445–9.

39. Lutz K, Yeoh KM, Macdermid JC, et al. Complications associated with operative versus nonsurgical treatment of distal radius fractures in patients aged 65 years and older. J Hand Surg Am 2014;39(7):1280–6.

40. Chung KC, Malay S, Shauver MJ, et al. Assessment of distal radius fracture complications among adults 60 years or older: a secondary analysis of the WRIST randomized clinical trial. JAMA Netw Open 2019;2(1):e187053.

41. McKay SD, MacDermid JC, Roth JH, et al. Assessment of complications of distal radius fractures and development of a complication checklist. J Hand Surg Am 2001;26(5):916–22.

42. Diaz-Garcia RJ, Oda T, Shauver MJ, et al. A systematic review of outcomes and complications of treating unstable distal radius fractures in the elderly. J Hand Surg Am 2011;36(5):824–35.e2.

43. Bruyere A, Vernet P, Botero SS, et al. Conservative treatment of distal fractures after the age of 65: a review of literature. Eur J Orthop Surg Traumatol 2018;28(8):1469–75.

44. Bartl C, Stengel D, Bruckner T, et al. Therapie der dislozierten intraartikulären distalen Radiusfraktur des älteren Patienten: Randomisierte Multicenterstudie (ORCHID) zur offenen Reposition und volaren Plattenosteosynthese versus geschlossener Reposition und Gipsimmobilisierung. Dtsch Arztebl Int 2014;111(46):779–87.

45. Chung KC, Malay S, Shauver MJ. Wrist and radius injury surgical trial group. the relationship between hand therapy and long-term outcomes after distal radius fracture in older adults: evidence from the randomized wrist and radius injury surgical trial. Plast Reconstr Surg 2019;144(2):230e–7e.

Closed Reduction Techniques for Distal Radius Fractures and Appropriate Casting Methods

Ashley B. Anderson, MD, Scott M. Tintle, MD, CDR MC USN*

KEYWORDS

• Distal radius fracture • Closed management • Reduction technique

KEY POINTS

• Distal radius fracture is one of the most common orthopedic injuries, and indications for closed management techniques should be understood.
• The goal of nonoperative management of distal radius fracture treatment is restoration of alignment and maintenance of the reduction.
• The maintenance of alignment is the key in determining whether a fracture is amenable to conservative management with closed reduction. Close follow-up is necessary to ensure alignment is maintained.

OVERVIEW AND RATIONALE

The goal of distal radius fracture treatment is to restore an upper extremity that has acceptable alignment, stability, and eventually mobility.[1] Although these fractures are common and often reviewed, there remains little evidence in supporting different treatment options.[2] Despite a lack of consensus, there continues to be an increase in the frequency of open reduction and internal fixation of distal radius fractures.[3] Despite this trend, closed reduction and immobilization in a cast remains an accepted and often the appropriate method of treatment of many distal radius fractures.

TREATMENT DECISION MAKING

The treatment of distal radius fractures practice guideline was approved by the American Academy of Orthopaedic Surgeons (AAOS) on December 4, 2009. The purpose of the Clinical Practice Guideline is to help improve treatment based on the current best available evidence.[2,4] When dealing with the treatment algorithm for distal radius fractures, the process begins with the decision as to whether or not it can be treated conservatively (closed manipulation and cast immobilization) or if it needs surgery. The goals of conservative management are to obtain and then subsequently maintain anatomic reduction in order to allow the fracture to heal with acceptable alignment with articular congruity. Patient and radiographic factors must be taken into consideration when selecting the best treatment options. Several important patient factors include patient age, bone quality, comorbidities, and occupation, whereas radiographic factors include fracture pattern and associated injuries. The basic parameter used to determine if a fracture is amenable to conservative management with closed reduction is if it will remain stable after reduction.

Department of Orthopaedic Surgery, Walter Reed National Military Medical Center, 8901 Rockville Pike, Bethesda, MD 20089, USA
* Corresponding author.
E-mail address: scott.tintle@gmail.com

Hand Clin 37 (2021) 239–245
https://doi.org/10.1016/j.hcl.2021.02.006
0749-0712/21/© 2021 Elsevier Inc. All rights reserved.

CLOSED TREATMENT MANAGEMENT
Indications

Assessment of postreduction stability is important in navigating distal radius fracture management. A stable fracture is one that is acceptably aligned after reduction and one with a low likelihood of postreduction displacement. Postreduction the position of the fracture fragments is maintained in the cast by soft tissue tension. Therefore, the prereduction findings, such as the initial fracture displacement, comminution, and impaction, are most important to recognize because these factors in combination cause fracture settling (leading to poor maintenance of length, rotation, and alignment) despite proper splinting and cast techniques. Fracture stability is best understood by identification of features that make a fracture unstable. In 1959, Lidstrom[5] found that a dorsal angulation exceeding 20° and 3 mm to 6 mm of radial shortening had a negative impact on patient function. These results are supported by Frykman (1967),[6] who used the same radiographic and similar clinical criteria. More recently, Lichtman and colleagues[7] discussed the AAOS Clinical Practice Guideline for managing distal radius fractures. There were only 5 moderate strength recommendations. These included

1. Surgical fixation for fractures that had a postreduction radial shortening greater than 3 mm, dorsal tilt greater than 10°, and intra-articular step-off greater than 2 mm
2. Rigid immobilization for nonoperative treatment
3. Use of a true lateral to assess the distal radioulnar joint
4. Initiation of early range of motion of the wrist after stable fixation
5. Use of vitamin C to help mitigate intractable pain[7]

With regard to conservative management, LaFontaine and colleagues[8] described fracture patterns at high risk for secondary displacement, despite acceptable postreduction and proper splinting. Fractures with 3 or more of the following are considered unstable and warrant close follow-up:

1. Having initial radiographs with more than 20° of dorsal (or palmar) angulation
2. A displacement of more than two-thirds the width of the shaft in any direction
3. Metaphyseal comminution

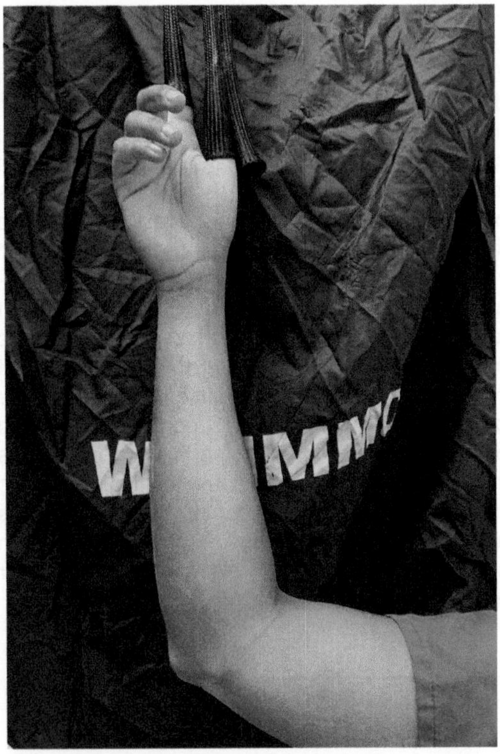

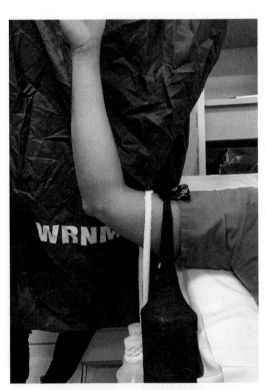

Fig. 1. Traction applied to the distal radius fracture typically is tolerated relatively well by patients, especially after providing a hematoma block.

Fig. 2. Weight applied to the arm. Gauze dressing bandage and saline bottles or stockinette and saline bottles make ideal weight for traction on the arm.

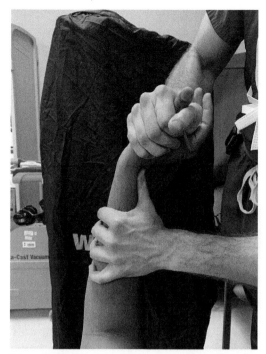

Fig. 3. This series of photos demonstrates the common maneuver to reduce the standard dorsally displaced distal radius fracture. Careful protection of fragile skin is necessary to prevent skin tears and degloving injuries.

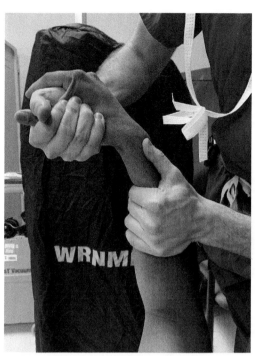

Fig. 5. To perform the reduction then pull traction to aid in carpal translation and push the distal distal fragment from dorsal to volar.

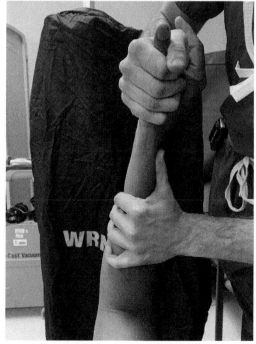

Fig. 4. To prepare for the reduction place one hand over the thenar eminence to pull traction and the thumb of the other hand on the dorsal edge of the distal fracture fragment.

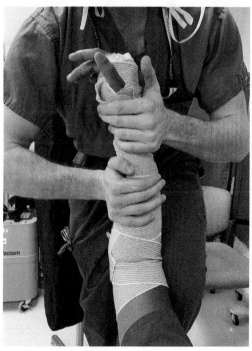

Fig. 6. Application of a 3-point mold. The mold can be applied with the flat part of the palm (see **Fig. 5**) or over the thigh of the surgeon (see Fig. 6).

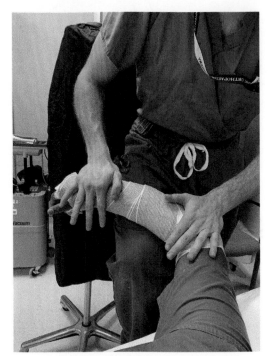

Fig. 7. Application of a 3-point mold. The mold can be applied with the flat part of the palm (see **Fig. 5**) or over the thigh of the surgeon (see **Fig. 6**).

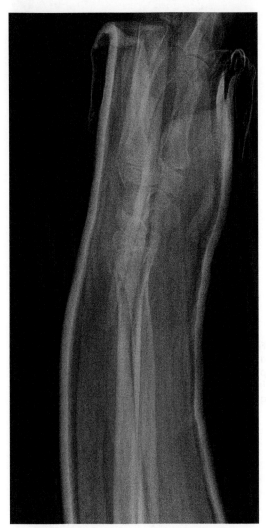

Fig. 9. Lateral radiograph status post–closed reduction with sugar tong splint application 3-point mold.

4. More than 5 mm of shortening
5. Intra-articular involvement
6. An associated ulna fracture
7. Advanced osteoporosis[8]

There is little consensus regarding the appropriate treatment of unstable distal radius fractures in elderly patients. Many studies of this patient population, including the randomized controlled Wrist and Radius Injury Surgical Trial,[9] have reported no difference in functional outcomes when patients whose age is greater than 60 are treated with closed reduction versus operatively for unstable fractures.[9–11]

In general, when determining the treatment plan, the following fractures are treated nonoperatively: (1) isolated extra-articular and (2) intra-articular with acceptable alignment and stability.[12]

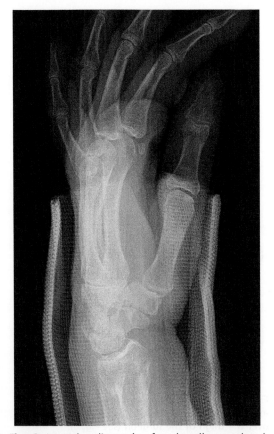

Fig. 8. Lateral radiograph of a dorsally angulated distal radius fracture before reduction.

Nondisplaced Fractures

Distal radius fractures that present with little to no displacement (<5° dorsal tilt and/or shortening less than 2 mm) have good long-term functional outcomes and prognosis when treated with nonoperative management with ACE wrap and/or splinting.[4] Of note, 1 complication associated with closed management of nondisplaced distal radius fractures includes spontaneous rupture of the extensor pollicis longus (EPL) tendon. These injuries usually occur within the first 2 months after sustaining a distal radius fracture and are thought to be due to the hypovascularity of EPL where Lister tubercle serves as a pulley for the tendon.[13–15]

Displaced Fractures

Closed reduction is the initial step for all displaced distal radius fractures. Closed reduction and splinting also can be considered, however, as a definitive treatment option when there is radiographic evidence that a stable realignment of the fracture fragments can be achieved, there are less than 3 of the Lafontaine criteria,[8] and residual interfragmentary fracture motion can be controlled with proper immobilization.

CLOSED REDUCTION
Anesthesia

The first step in closed reduction is to provide analgesia with a hematoma block. Inject a local anesthetic through the skin of the dorsal wrist directly into the fracture site. Aspiration of a subtle blush into the syringe plunger confirms location in the fracture hematoma prior to injection. In order to make this step more pleasant for the patient, a small wheal of lidocaine can be injected in the subcutaneous tissue 5 minutes prior to the hematoma block.

Traction

In preparation for a reduction maneuver, the patient can be placed in finger traps for multiplanar ligamentotaxis for approximately 10 minutes.[16] The patient's index and thumb are suspended by finger traps with 10 lb of traction applied to the arm by hanging 10 lb over the elbow positioned at 90° of flexion. It is critical to be cognizant of the patient's skin examination and quality. Skin tears are more common in the elderly patient population.[17] During traction, anteroposterior/lateral traction radiographs can be obtained to provide information about intra-articular fragments similar to computed tomography[18,19] but at lower cost[20] (**Figs. 1** and **2**).

Manual Reduction

Reduction is obtained by supination, traction, midcarpal extension, and anterior transplant of the distal fracture fragment.[12] Radial length is restored by traction alone. The palmar translation of the hand relative to the distal radius in combination with pronation of the hand relative to the wrist restores palmar tilt and radial inclination[21] (**Figs. 3–5**).

Immobilization

Postreduction, the extremity is immobilized in a splint with appropriate 3-point mold for approximately 7 days to 10 days[1,12] to accommodate for soft tissue swelling. In a dorsally displaced fracture pattern, the 3-point model holds the postreduction alignment, through tension across the dorsoradial soft tissue hinge from slight flexion and ulnar deviation of the hand. Position of immobilization for a dorsally angulated distal radius fractures involving the metaphysis is neutral to slight flexion, 20° to 30° of ulnar deviation with neutral forearm rotation[22] (**Figs. 6** and **7**).

The sugar tong splint is the most commonly used splint after reduction because the above-elbow splint prevents rotation of the forearm.[23] One large prospective, randomized study found no difference in redisplacement risk (sugar tong

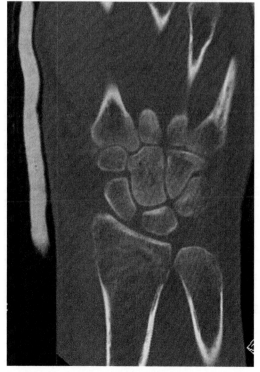

Fig. 10. Coronal slice of computed tomography scan demonstrating near anatomic reduction.

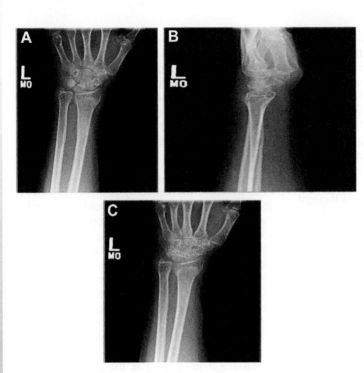

Fig. 11. (*A*) PA, (*B*) lateral, and (*C*) oblique radiographs demonstrate shortening of the radius but overall alignment is maintained.

splint vs radial gutter splint) and that radial gutter splints can lead to increased patient satisfaction and comfort.[24] Splint choice varies by physician preference. In general, the splint should be well padded without wrinkles in the plaster or soft-cotton roll, and it should end proximal to the metacarpal heads at the level of the distal palmar crease to allow finger range of motion to prevent stiffness.

After splint immobilization is completed, the patient is transitioned to a short arm cast with a good 3-point mold for approximately 3 weeks to 6 weeks, with radiographs obtained at weekly intervals to monitor fracture alignment.[1] It is imperative to compare the follow-up radiographs to the initial postreduction radiographs to observe true changes in alignment.[12] After 3 weeks, typically a patient's follow-up is spaced out until the 6-week time frame, because surgery is not likely at that time. Once there is radiographic evidence of healing with fracture callus, the patient should begin wrist range-of-motion exercises promptly. These occur routinely at approximately 6 weeks after closed reduction (**Figs. 8–11**).

SUMMARY

Stable, distal radius fractures may be treated with conservative management by restoration of length, rotation, and alignment through closed reduction and splinting. After a period of immobilization, patients should undergo formal physical therapy. It is imperative surgeons assess distal radius fracture stability accurately and exercise proper techniques for successful nonoperative management of distal radius fractures.

ACKNOWLEDGMENT

We would like to thank Dr. Matthew J. Kinnard, MD for his assistance in obtaining clinical photographs for this work.

DISCLOSURE

The views expressed are those of the author and do not reflect the official policy of the Department of the Army/Navy/Air Force, Department of Defense, or US Government.

REFERENCES

1. Schneppendahl J, Windolf J, Kaufmann RA. Distal radius fractures: current concepts. J Hand Surg 2012;37(8):1718–25.
2. Hammert WC, Kramer RC, Graham B, et al. AAOS appropriate use criteria: treatment of distal radius fractures. J Am Acad Orthop Surg 2013;21(8):506–9.
3. Mattila VM, Huttunen TT, Sillanpää P, et al. Significant change in the surgical treatment of distal radius fractures: a nationwide study between 1998 and 2008 in finland. J Trauma 2011;71(4):939–43.
4. Murray J, Gross L. Treatment of distal radius fractures. J Am Acad Orthop Surg 2013;21(8):502–5.

5. Lidstrom A. Fractures of the distal end of the radius. A clinical and statistical study of end results. Acta Orthop Scand Suppl 1959;41:1–118.

6. Frykman G. Fracture of the distal radius including sequelae-shoulder–handfinger syndrome, disturbance in the distal radio-ulnar joint and impairment of nerve function: a clinical and experimental study. Acta Orthop Scand 2014;38(sup108):1–61.

7. Lichtman DM, Bindra RR, Boyer MI, et al. Treatment of distal radius fractures. J Am Acad Orthop Surg 2010;18(3):180–9.

8. Lafontaine M, Hardy D, Delince P. Stability assessment of distal radius fractures. Injury 1989;20(4):208–10.

9. Chung KC, Kim HM, Malay S, et al. The wrist and radius injury surgical trial (WRIST): 12-month outcomes from a multicenter international randomized clinical trial. Plast Reconstr Surg 2020;1. https://doi.org/10.1097/prs.0000000000006829.

10. Ju J-H, Jin G-Z, Li G-X, et al. Comparison of treatment outcomes between nonsurgical and surgical treatment of distal radius fracture in elderly: a systematic review and meta-analysis. Langenbecks Arch Surg 2015;400(7):767–79.

11. Diaz-Garcia RJ, Oda T, Shauver MJ, et al. A systematic review of outcomes and complications of treating unstable distal radius fractures in the elderly. J Hand Surg 2011;36(5):824–35.e2.

12. Eglseder WA. Atlas of Upper Extremity Trauma, A Clinical Perspective. 1st Ed. Springer; 2018.

13. Cooney WP, Dobyns JH, Linscheid RL. Complications of Colles' fractures. J Bone Joint Surg Am 1980;62(4):613–9.

14. Helal B, Chen SC, Iwegbu G. Rupture of the extensor pollicis longus tendon in undisplaced colles' type of fracture. Hand (N Y) 1982;os-14(1):41–7.

15. Weinberg ED. Late spontaneous rupture of the extensor pollicis longus tendon following colles' fracture. J Am Med Assoc 1950;142(13):979.

16. Agee JM. Distal radius fractures. Multiplanar ligamentotaxis. Hand Clin 1993;9(4):577–85.

17. Levin LS, Rozell JC, Pulos N. Distal radius fractures in the elderly. J Am Acad Orthop Surg 2017;25(3):179–87.

18. Harness NG, Ring D, Zurakowski D, et al. The influence of three-dimensional computed tomography reconstructions on the characterization and treatment of distal radial fractures. J Bone Joint Surg Am 2006;88(6):1315–23.

19. Katz MA, Beredjiklian PK, Bozentka DJ, et al. Computed tomography scanning of intra-articular distal radius fractures: does it influence treatment? J Hand Surg 2001;26(3):415–21.

20. Goldwyn E, Pensy R, O'Toole RV, et al. Do traction radiographs of distal radial fractures influence fracture characterization and treatment? J Bone Joint Surg Am 2012;94(22):2055–62.

21. Dée W, Klein W, Rieger H. Reduction techniques in distal radius fractures. Injury 2000;31:48–55.

22. Wolfe SW, Hotchkiss RN, Pederson WC, et al. Green's operative hand surgery. 7th edition. Elsevier; 2011.

23. Diaz-Garcia RJ, Chung KC. Common myths and evidence in the management of distal radius fractures. Hand Clin 2012;28(2):127–33.

24. Bong MR, Egol KA, Leibman M, et al. A comparison of immediate postreduction splinting constructs for controlling initial displacement of fractures of the distal radius: a prospective randomized study of long-arm versus short-arm splinting. J Hand Surg 2006;31(5):766–70.

Kirschner Wire Fixation of Distal Radius Fractures, Indication, Technique and Outcomes

Michael B. Gottschalk, MD[a],*, Eric R. Wagner, MD, MS[b,c]

KEYWORDS

- Kirschner wire • Closed reduction and percutaneous pinning (CRPP) • Distal radius • Fracture

KEY POINTS

- Percutaneous pin fixation of distal radius fractures is a viable option in extra-articular and simple intra-articular fractures.
- Early techniques have been improved on to capture various fragments that initially were under-recognized.
- Common complications include loss of reduction and superficial infection.
- Currently, there is no consensus on the treatment of distal radius fractures as it relates to closed reduction and percutaneous pin versus open reduction and internal fixation.

EPIDEMIOLOGY

Distal radius fractures comprise approximately 44% of all upper extremity fractures that present to the emergency department in the United States.[1] Studies show that fractures occur in a bimodal distribution involving children in their first and second decades of life and adults in their sixth and seventh decades.[2] In addition to age, both sex and ethnicity also have been shown to have a propensity for increased risk of fracture, with white women involved in up to 83% of adult cases.[2] Because distal radius fractures occur among such a wide demographic spectrum, it should come as no surprise that there is a plethora of treatment modalities employed in the care of distal radius fractures. This article focuses specifically on the indications, technique, and outcomes of Kirschner (K)-wire fixation for distal radius fractures.

INDICATIONS/CONTRAINDICATIONS
Operative Treatment Indications

The surgical treatment of distal radius fractures has been increasing since the early 2000s.[3] This increased incidence of surgically treated fractures is multifactorial, with marketing, technology, and evidenced-based practices contributing to the rise. In 2009, the American Academy of Orthopaedic Surgeons (AAOS) put out Clinical Practice Guidline (CPGs) for the treatment of distal radius fractures. The CPG recommended operative intervention in patients who had radial shortening by greater than 3 mm, dorsal tilt of greater than 10°, and an intra-articular step-off of greater than 2 mm. This recommendation received a moderate rating whereas most others received an inconclusive ranking.

Much of the controversy stems from the difficulty in discerning those fractures that are

[a] Department of Orthopaedics, Division of Plastic Surgery, Emory School of Medicine, Atlanta Veteran Affairs Hospital, Grady Memorial Hospital, Morehouse School of Medicine, 59 Executive Park Drive South, Atlanta, GA 30329, USA; [b] Department of Orthopaedics, Division of Plastic Surgery, Emory School of Medicine, Grady Memorial Hospital, Morehouse School of Medicine, 59 Executive Park Drive South, Atlanta, GA 30329, USA; [c] Emory Orthopaedics and Spine Center, 59 Executive Park Drive South, Atlanta, GA 30329, USA
* Corresponding author.
E-mail address: michael.gottschalk@emoryhealthcare.org

Hand Clin 37 (2021) 247–258
https://doi.org/10.1016/j.hcl.2021.02.007

unstable and at risk for loss of reduction with closed means. A radiographic study by Lafontaine and colleagues[4] reviewed 112 cases treated by closed means that evaluated variables for risk of loss of reduction. The investigators concluded that dorsal angulation greater than 20°, dorsal comminution, intra-articular radiocarpal fracture, associated ulnar fracture, and age over 60 years old were strong predictors for loss of initial reduction.[4] Several studies have tried to corroborate or expound on these variables.[5,6] LaMartina and colleagues[6] reviewed more than 168 fractures in an effort to validate Lafontaine and colleagues' criteria and Margaret McQueen's formula. Ultimately, the investigators concluded that both prior articles had good predictability for final radial height, inclination, and ulnar variance but that each failed to predict ultimate dorsal tilt. LaMartina and colleagues'[6] study demonstrated that the ability to "hook" the volar cortex during the initial reduction was most predictive in the overall final volar tilt. This parameter, in conjunction with LaFontaine and colleagues and McQueen, often are used to help justify the use of operative techniques (**Table 1**).

Indications for Closed Reduction and Percutaneous Pin in Adult Patients

Although there are no absolute indications for the usage of K-wires for distal radius fractures over other treatment modalities, several soft indications remain present owing to the practicality of the treatment. For instance, most physicians agree that extra-articular fractures (eg, Orthopedic Trauma Association/Association for Osteosynthesis AO/OTA) or those with minimal articular step-off that are reducible via ligamentotaxis may undergo CRPP or nonoperative management.

Dorsally displaced fractures are the most ideal pattern for CRPP, given the potential location and placement of K-wires dorsally to hold the reduction. Despite the K-wires being placed dorsally, several structures remain at risk. Santoshi and colleagues[7] performed a cadaveric distal radius model by placing several common K-wires about the wrist, then dissecting out the closest structures to the K-wires. The most commonly reported structures at risk were extensor tendons to the fingers and thumb as well as superficial branch of the radial nerve (SBRN).[7] Despite the relative risk to these structures, it is implicit that dorsally placed K-wires are preferred over volar wires, owing to the risk to the major volar neurovascular structures (ie, the median and ulnar nerves and the radial and ulnar arteries) and the flexor tendons of the digits. As such, fractures that are dorsally displaced lend themselves to treatment by closed means with K-wire fixation.

Indications for Closed Reduction and Percutaneous Pin in Pediatric Patients

Pediatric fractures with open physes often are treated best via closed means or with supplemental K-wire fixation (**Fig. 1**). K-wire fixation is preferred due primarily to the risk of growth plate injuries with internal hardware (eg plates/screws) and the high propensity for hardware complications.[8] A meta-analysis by Sengab and colleagues primarily reviewed 6 articles regarding the risk of redisplacement after closed treatment and casting versus the addition of K-wire fixation in children. Although K-wire fixation reduced the risk of loss of reduction significantly, from 45.7% to 3.8%, the overall functional outcome did not change by treatment modality.[8] Thus, the investigators concluded that a wide range of reductions may be tolerated in children owing to their remodeling potential. Unfortunately, long-term outcomes are lacking and it is possible that continued pain or dysfunction in adolescence or adulthood may ensue. Ultimately, it is important to consider a patient's age, time to skeletal maturity, and type of fracture when deciding the optimal treatment choice.

Table 1
Predictors of nonoperative loss of reduction of distal radius fractures

Reference	Radial Shortening	Dorsal Tilt	Articular Step-off	Ulnar Fracture	Dorsal Comminution	Age	Hook Volar Cortex
LaFontaine and colleagues[4]		>20°		Yes	Yes	>60 y	
McQueen and colleagues[5]				Yes, ulnar variance	Yes, metaphyseal	Yes	
LaMartina and colleagues[6]							Yes
AAOS CPG	>3 mm	>10°	>2 mm				

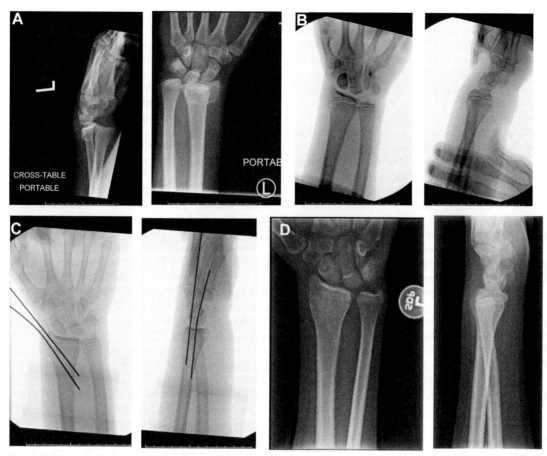

Fig. 1. (*A*) This is a depiction of a 17-year-old boy with open physes and a dorsally displaced distal radius fracture. (*B*) Demonstrates a closed reduction of the fracture with adequate alignment. (*C*) Demonstrates the use of 2 radial styloid K-wires as mirrored after Mah and Atkinson. (*D*) Demonstrates the postoperative radiographs on follow-up with adequate healing in acceptable alignment.

Classification Schemes

As with all fractures, delineating the type and understanding the nuances of different displacement forces are essential to discerning which treatment modality best serves the patient. Several classification systems have been utilized over the years, including the following: an eponym-based system (eg, Colles, Smith, and Barton), Lidström, Castaing and Le Club, Older, Sarmiento, Melone, Jenkins, AO/OTA/Association for the Study of Internal Fixation [ASIF], Mayo, McMurtry, Fernandez, Universal, Mathoulin, and Shin and Schenck.[9] Although several classification system schema are available, few are helpful in determining the ultimate treatment modality needed.

Contraindications to Closed Reduction and Percutaneous Pin

Although there are few absolute contraindications to the usage of K-wire fixation in distal radius

fractures, there are several instances in which treatment with K-wires may portend a poor outcome. Patients with significant osteoporotic bone, concomitant open wounds, or fractures with a shear component (eg, Barton fracture or OTA type B fractures) or significant intra-articular component (eg, OTA type C fractures) are best treated primarily with other techniques. For instance, patients with osteoporotic bone may best be treated with a dorsal spanning plate and adjuvant K-wires as opposed to K-wires alone.

TECHNIQUE/PROCEDURAL APPROACH

Drs Diaz-Garcia and Chung[10] have written a historical treatise on the evolution of treatments ranging from Colles' nonoperative management in 1814 to the earliest reports of operative intervention in the 1900s. This article is a comprehensive historical synopsis of the various time periods of significant scientific advancement in the treatment of distal radius fractures. One such time period, the Era of Refinement, denotes the time period from 1965 to the present and represents a collection of techniques that scholars have advanced over time through scrutiny and innovation. During this era, CRPP dominated much of the initial treatments.

One important consideration when considering CRPP is to understand the various decisions that must be made before undertaking a trip to the operating room. Dr John Rayhack[11] eloquently described the various historical techniques and the considerations made prior to percutaneous pinning of the distal radius. The most important considerations include those that relate to the pins, reduction maneuvers, postoperative immobilization, and intraoperative radiographic techniques. In regard to the pins, it is important to think about size and number (Table 2), threaded or nonthreaded, location and angle of insertion, insertion technique (ie, power or manual), percutaneous or open placement, need for removal (eg, pins out of skin or cut under skin), and the duration of pinning.[11] Although studies have looked at several these variables, the main focus of this section is to discuss the number, location, and insertion angles of various K-wires.

Historical Techniques of Closed Reduction and Percutaneous Pin

Lambotte published the first initial report on using K-wires for the treatment of distal radius fractures in 1908.[12] His surgical technique placed a single K-wire through the radial styloid in an oblique orientation across the fracture site. This technique later was reported on by several physicians expounding on more than 150 surgical cases and their relevant complications.[13–16] These are denoted in (Table 3). In 1992, Mah and Atkinson[17] refined the procedure by adding a second K-wire to control rotational stability of the fracture (Fig. 2). These techniques are best employed for extra-articular fractures where there is no dorsal

ulnar fracture fragment that may cause a loss of reduction.

In 1952, DePalma[18] attempted to decrease the rate of fracture displacement in more comminuted distal radius fractures by using the ulna to keep the radius length stable. He reported a case series of 28 comminuted distal radius fractures that underwent ulnar-radial pinning sparing the distal radioulnar joint (DRUJ).[18] The specific technique describes a threaded K-wire inserted 4 cm proximal from the ulnar styloid at a 45o angle aimed toward the radial styloid (see Fig. 2). As with other techniques, using a single K-wire for complex fractures resulted in several complications, including loss of reduction, pin migration, and infection (see Table 3).

It was not until 1975 that Stein and Katz[19] would consider placing 2 K-wires in different planes to capture various fragments about the distal radius. The investigators described a technique whereby a K-wire was inserted through the radial styloid in addition to the dorsal ulnar corner of the distal radius (see Fig. 2). The most common complications related to this type of fixation method were skin-related issues from the K-wires and prolonged immobilization of the fractures.

In 1976, Uhl described a slightly different technique whereby a radial styloid K-wire still was placed, but the second K-wire instead was placed through the ulna and DRUJ and into the distal radius itself (see Fig. 2). For this technique to be employed, it is imperative that the ulnar–to-radial pin capture the fracture fragments. Table 3 delineates the various other case series that reported on this technique and the ensuing complications.

At the same time Uhl was presenting his technique, Kapandji[20] introduced a new method of buttressing the fracture, called intrafocal pinning. In 1976, he described using 2 pins through the fracture site to buttress the fracture volarly (see Fig. 2). This technique later changed to using 3 K-wires.[21] Over the next 15 years, more than 7 different articles would be published elucidating the various complications in hundreds of patients (see Table 3). Despite the rapid assimilation of this technique into practice, there still were significant complications, including a high rate of loss of reduction/fracture displacement and significant tendon irritation.

In an effort to improve on prior results, Dr Rayhack and colleagues[22] first published their technique of multiplanar ulna-to-radius pinning with fixation of the DRUJ in 1989. This technique is accomplished by using a traction device to obtain the reduction of the wrist and then placing a series of K-wires from the ulna to the radius, starting distally across the DRUJ in a transverse fashion

Table 2 Kirschner wire sizes	
Size (in)	Size (mm)
.028	0.7
.035	0.9
.045	1.1
.054	1.4
.062	1.6

Table 3
Historical techniques for closed reduction and percutaneous of distal radius fractures with their reported complications

Year	Surgeon	Technique	Depiction	Case Report Number	Complications
Radial styloid pin (1 pin [Lambott] or 2 pins [Mah and Alkinson] drilled through radial styloid slightly divergent)					
1908	Lambotte	Single radial styloid pin			
1959	Willenegger and Guggenbuhl	Lambott		25	5 Sudeck atrophies; 3 redisplacements; 3 inadequate reductions; failure rate of 18%
1965	Buzyn	Lambott variant		132	28% secondary fracture displacement
1982	Docquier	Lambott		32	
1983	Freising and Walter	Lambott			
1986	Kerboul	Lambott		32	1 redisplacement; 5 pain dysfunctions (troubles tophiques); 2 tendon irritations; 2 SBRNs; 2 infections
1992	Mah and Atkinson	Two radial styloid pins	Figure	32	
Ulnar-radial pinning without fixation of the DRUJ 45° 4 cm proximal to the ulnar styloid drilled to the radial styloid					
1952	DePalma	Ulnar-radial fixation	Figure	28	2 infections
1961	Dowling and Sawyer	DePalma		51	7 poor pin placements; less than optimal in 15; loss of reduction in 7; 2 broken pins; 5 small finger MCP contractures; 1 CRPS
1969	Ledoux et al	Depalma		24	11 failed reductions/redisplacements
Radial styloid pinning and dorsal pinning					
1975	Stein and Katz	Single radial styloid and dorsal ulnar pin	Figure	37	7 pins eroded through the skin (initially buried under the skin); 1 tenolysis of FPL due to pin migration; 1 Sudeck atrophy
1984	Clancy			30	13/30 returned to operating room for pin removal
1990	Kwasny			47	1 Sudeck atrophy

(continued on next page)

Table 3
(continued)

Year	Surgeon	Technique	Depiction	Case Report Number	Complications
Radial styloid and ulnar-radial pinning of the posteromedial fragment					
1976	Uhl	Radial styloid pin, ulnar to radial DRUJ pin	Figure		
1982	Lortat-Jacob			17	1 CRPS; 1 SBRN; and no fracture redisplacement
1983	Mortier			42	2 fracture displacements; sympathetic dystrophy in 3 patients; carpal tunnel syndrome in 1 patient
1986	Mortier			68	Expanded series from 1983
Kapandji double and triple intrafocal pinning to the fracture surface					
1976	Kapandji	Double pinning	Figure		
1987	Kapandji	Triple pinning			
1982	Epinette	Double pinning		72	
1982	Dockquier			32	
1986	Kerboul			30	Loss of reduction; extensor tendon rupture; SBRN, RSD; early pin removal; fracture displacement postponing; and infection
1987	Peyroux			159	
1987	Nonnemacher and Neumeier			150	
1988	Nonnemacher and Kempf	2-pin and 3-pin technique		350	
1991	Greatting	3-pin technique		60	
Ulnar-radial pinning with fixation of the DRUJ 4-9 K-wires inserted ulnar to radial at various angles					
1989	Rayhack	Ulnar-radial pinning	Figure	14	
1991	Rayhack			27	4 pin breakages; 1 pin migration; 1 loss of reduction; 3 patients with flexion lag

Abbreviations: MCP, metacarpophalangeal; RSD, reflex sympathetic dystrophy.

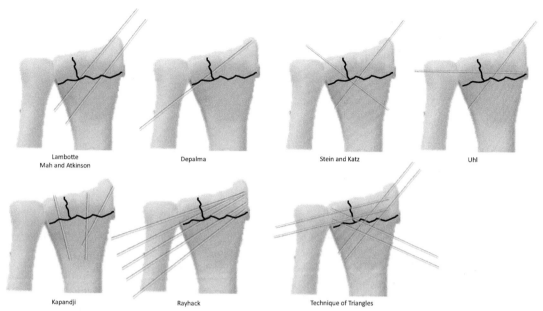

Fig. 2. Compilation of techniques as described from historical perspectives with the appropriate eponym associated with each technique.

and moving to most proximal with a more angled trajectory (see **Fig. 2**). In a series of 14 patients, they only had a few who demonstrated loss of reduction or pin breakage, with the vast majority doing well with near-full pronation and supination despite having fixation across the DRUJ.

Recent Techniques of Closed Reduction and Percutaneous Pin

A full account of all studies published on these various techniques is located in **Table 3**, with their denoted complications when available. Newer techniques using percutaneous K-wire fixation have been published, but most incorporate the principles from the historic articles. One such recent article by Vidyadharan[23] creates a triangular configuration combining several of the techniques, including ulnar-radial pinning across the DRUJ, 2 K-wires through the radial styloid, and an additional 2 K-wires from the radius into the dorsal ulnar fragment (see **Fig. 2**). This technique was tested in 108 individuals with OTA type B and type C fractures ranging from ages 18 to 84. The author demonstrated 87% excellent or good results. Comparison to other methods was not attempted, however, and long-term results and complications were indeterminate.

Despite the extensive volume of publications on various techniques and their relative complications, the AAOS 2009 CPG had a consensus statement that the number of K-wires needed for CRPP of the distal radius currently is inconclusive. This

likely is related to the large number of fracture patterns encountered and the multitude of CRPP techniques currently available for treatment of these injuries.

Previously, investigators have documented the relative trends in treatment as they have evolved over time.[3,24,25] Despite a robust body of literature demonstrating reasonable outcomes, the incidence of CRPP performed has varied widely across training types,[25] with little recorded rationale available to explain its rapid decline.[24] As part of an American Board of Orthopaedic Surgery (ABOS) project, the authors previously reviewed all distal radius cases presented to the ABOS for certification for part II of the physician board certification. The study identified a decline in CRPP usage from 20% in 2007 to 15% of operatively treated fractures by orthopedic surgery board applicants in 2013.[26] **Fig. 3** demonstrates this linear incline of volar plate usage at the expense of CRPP and external fixation.

RECOVERY AND REHABILITATION

The postoperative course for patients undergoing CRPP can vary substantially. Significant controversy exists regarding the timing of K-wire removal and the type of postoperative orthosis used.

Immobilization Type

Currently, there is no level I evidence that has demonstrated superiority of any specific type of

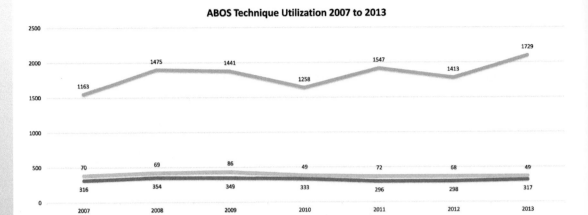

Fig. 3. ABOS incline of rates of ORIF as opposed to CRPP and external fixation, from 2007 to 2013.

immobilization following distal radius fractures treated either nonoperatively or operatively.[27–30] The current options studied include radial gutter, ulnar gutter, sugar tong, short arm, and long arm splints/casts. When comparing most historic types of K-wire techniques, including Lambotte, Uhl, Stein and Katz, and Rayhack, most of the initial articles had large variations in the type of postoperative immobilization utilized. As such, drawing comparisons between K-wire configurations is made more difficult, given the extra variable of type of postoperative immobilization.[11] Therefore, as a gestalt, immobilizing only the injured joint is recommended in an effort to prevent postoperative stiffness in adjacent joints, except for when the DRUJ also may be involved. Most recently, Caruso and colleagues[31] evaluated 74 patients with closed reduction and cast immobilization in either a short arm or long arm cast cohort. Radiographic evaluation occurred at 7 days to 10 days, 4 weeks, and 12 weeks. The investigators found no statistically significant difference across cohorts for any variable nor was there any correlation with clinical patient-reported outcomes. The only statistically significant finding was improved Mayo elbow scores in patients who did not have their elbow immobilized during their short-term follow-up. In a biomechanical study, Rahman and colleagues[32] evaluated the biomechanical rotational stability afforded by 4 different immobilization constructs. The investigators demonstrated that involving more proximal structures in the orthosis utilized demonstrated better rotational control (eg, Muenster over short arm cast). Further immobilization proximal to the epicondyles, however, did not provide further stabilization. Expert opinion thus advises immobilizing patients based on stability of the fracture, stability of the K-wire construct, stability of the DRUJ, and potential location for instability.

Removal of the Kirschner Wires

Similar to the method of immobilization, the timing of the removal of K-wires associated with CRPP of distal radius fractures is variable. One of the most feared complications of CRPP is the development of infections and stiffness of the joint. A report by Strickland and colleagues[33] on phalangeal fractures demonstrated increased stiffness and risk for infection when K-wires were left in place past 4 weeks. This essentially has been extrapolated to other aspects of the hand and wrist. In certain instances, K-wires may be left in place for up to 6 weeks or 8 weeks, but there is a progressive increased risk of infection the longer the K-wires are left in place. Additionally, if the K-wires are buried under the skin, it may be possible to leave them in place longer and remove them either in an office setting under direct local anesthesia or in the operating room. One complication of burying the K-wires is erosion back through the skin, which can be painful for patients.

Preferred Method

The authors' preferred method of immobilization depends on a patient's bone quality, fracture reduction, and pin construct. For most patients, the authors use a circumferential short arm cast. In patients requiring more radial support, the authors utilize a radial gutter, including the index and middle fingers for added support, especially in pediatric patients. If a transulnar-to-radial pin is utilized, or if the distal ulna fracture is associated with DRUJ instability, the authors recommend the use of a sugar tong in an effort to prevent pin breakage at the DRUJ. K-wires are kept in place for 4 weeks to 6 weeks, with removal timing based on clinical and radiographic signs of fracture stability and healing. At 4 weeks, if radiographs demonstrate no evidence of shifting and the patient is nontender, the pins are removed in the office and the patient is placed in a removable brace. At 6 weeks, formal hand therapy is begun, focusing on range of motion while weaning from a thermoplastic splint over the following 2 weeks to 3 weeks.

OUTCOMES

There is a significant body of literature describing the outcomes following distal radius fractures treated with percutaneous pin fixation. There continues to be significant controversy, however, over which treatment offers superior results. In part, this can be explained by the large number of treatment types with significant variability within each technique, including number of K-wires, placement of K-wires, fracture type, postoperative immobilization, complications, and unique patient characteristics (eg, age). The initial historical data using percutaneous pin are summarized in **Table 3**, with the various complication rates depicted for each case series when available. This data are of limited use, given the relatively poor understanding of distal radius fractures during this time frame and the lack of standardization of reporting outcomes following surgical techniques. In recent years, level 1 and level 2 randomized controlled trials have compared different techniques while focusing on fracture type, patient-reported outcome measures, short-term and long-term temporal endpoints, and cost. When comparing the outcomes of percutaneous pin fixation for distal radius fractures, the other 2 most commonly performed treatments, including closed reduction and splinting and open reduction and internal fixation (ORIF) with volar-locked plating, must be accounted for.

Closed Reduction and Splinting Versus Percutaneous Pin Fixation

A recent meta-analysis performed by Karantana and colleagues[34] has reviewed the 26 available studies comparing various forms of CRPP to closed treatment and splinting/casting. Based on a heterogeneous population and the various methods for pinning and immobilization, there remain significant biases in any outcomes reported. This specific comparison was tested in 11 studies, with a total of 917 patients in dorsally displaced distal radius fractures. Nine of the 11 trials had K-wires that crossed the fracture site whereas 2 used Kapandji intrafocal pinning. Unfortunately, most of the trials did not note patient-reported outcome measures, limiting the ability to comment directly on the effect on this type of outcome. Fracture displacement

requiring secondary treatment following splinting without K-wire fixation occurred in 12% of patients whereas none in the percutaneous pinning group required intervention. In contrast, those treated with K-wires demonstrated a 7% infection rate requiring antibiotics in addition to early K-wire removal. The pinning cohort demonstrated a higher rate of complex regional pain syndrome (CRPS), although it is stipulated that this may be due to bias in a single study that showed a 28% rate of CRPS in the short term. In addition, there was a higher propensity for developing carpal tunnel syndrome in the nonoperative cohort (3.7%), which may be attributable to the position of the splint/cast. Ultimately, the investigators of the meta-analysis could not make any generalizable statement on radiologic outcomes, return to work, grip strength, or any physician-reported outcomes owing to the incompleteness of most studies.

Percutaneous Pin Fixation Versus Open Reduction and Internal Fixation with Volar-Locked Plating

Recent trends have demonstrated a significant increase in the use of volar-locked plating in the treatment of distal radius fractures.[3,25] As part of an ABOS study and follow-up to Koval and colleagues'[24] initial study, the authors investigated the trends of the treatment of distal radius fractures between 2007 and 2013.[24,26] Ultimately, Koval and colleagues' trend continued, showing that surgeons utilized CRPP approximately 15%, external fixation 2%, and ORIF more than 82%. In part, this likely is due to the training received during fellowship, perceived benefit and ease of technique with ORIF, and the strong marketing from implant companies.[25] Because of this large surge in open operative fixation, there have been more than 7 randomized control trials comparing CRPP to ORIF for distal radius fracture treatment within the past decade.[35–42] Although these studies can be examined independently, each study reported various individual findings likely biased by relatively lower numbers than a multicenter trial or meta-analysis.

Chaudhry and colleagues[43] performed a meta-analysis study with patients treated with CRPP and those with ORIF for AO/OTA types A, B, and C fractures. There were more type A fractures owing to the fact that several studies only reported on extra-articular dorsally displaced fractures. At 3 months, there were 414 patients with Disabilities of the Arm, Shoulder and Hand (DASH) follow-up in 6 of the randomized clinical trials (RCTs). The results demonstrated a 7.5 mean difference, with a CI between 4.4 and 10.6 (minimal clinically important difference [MCID] for DASH is 10[44]) in favor of volar-locked plating. Similarly, function at 6 months and at 12 months was reported with DASH scores in 875 patients in 7 RCTs and showed a mean difference of 3.8, with a CI between 1.2 and 6.3 in favor of volar-locked plating. Neither of these time points reached the MCID for DASH scores and, as such, it is unclear whether there is a clinical benefit during these follow-ups in regard to patient-reported outcomes. When comparing complications between the CRPP and ORIF cohorts, ORIF demonstrated fewer infections—14 (3.2%) versus 36 (8.2%) (P<.001), respectively. All other complications, including deep infection, neurologic injury, tendon rupture, and reoperations, were not statistically significant between the 2 groups. In addition, there was no statistical difference in radiologic outcomes as measured between the 2 groups. In light of these findings, the investigators noted that there was a slight improvement in DASH scores in those who received ORIF over CRPP of unknown significance. It is possible that earlier time points may show a bigger difference (eg, 6 weeks) due to the postoperative immobilization required by CRPP. At long-term follow-up, the cost increase of using a plate is not beneficial, although the argument for plate usage may be better realized in earlier time points due to quicker range of motion and return to work, as well as a lower infection rate.[45] Ultimately, surgeon discretion should be exercised to explain the pros and cons for each surgical intervention and the relevant associated complications.

COMPLICATIONS

Complications following distal radius fractures and the treatment of those complications have been well documented in the literature.[7,46,47] The following types of complications have been reported in the literature after CRPP of distal radius fracture: loss of reduction, tendon attrition/rupture, neurologic symptoms, hardware complication (eg, pin breakage or migration), DRUJ instability, vascular injury, and infection/hematoma.

In an effort to mitigate these complications, Santoshi and colleagues[7] performed a cadaveric study evaluating the proximity of different anatomic structures to various pin placements. The investigators demonstrated that the cephalic vein and the extensor tendons were among the most commonly injured structures, whereas the neurologic structures (eg, SBRN) were involved but to a lesser extent. It is possible, however, that the nerve's proximity to the K-wires can cause irritation to the nerve when the hand or wrist is moved. As such, the investigators recommended a small incision and spreading down to the bone

to avoid any inadvertent injuries while pinning. The authors' preferred technique is to penetrate the skin with the wire manually and then advance the K-wire on oscillation mode.

Long-term complications have been studied in patients who underwent CRPP compared with ORIF.[47] Liao and colleagues[47] reviewed reoperation rates during an 8-year period of patients who underwent CRPP versus volar-locked plating. The investigators included 1364 cases with approximately equal cohorts. The study demonstrated that the CRPP group had higher rates of revision surgery (P = .003). The overall reoperation rate was similar, however, between cohorts. This was secondary to other complications in the ORIF group, including tendon irritation, neurologic issues, and hardware irritation. The investigators concluded that the overall rate of reoperation was similar among the cohorts with a varying of the type of complication noted for each subset. Thus, it is necessary to counsel the patient on the type of fixation they may receive and what the perceived pros and cons are for that specific treatment.

CLINICS CARE POINTS

- Distal radius fractures comprise the largest portion of upper extremity fractures that report to the emergency department with a bimodal distribution peaking in their first and second as well as sixth and seventh decades of life.

- A comprehensive understanding of the fracture morphology is imperative when deciding which CRPP technique to use to reduce the risk of complications following surgical intervention.

- Indications for CRPP of distal radius fractures include extra-articular fractures with dorsal displacement, simple articular fractures that reduce with ligamentotaxis, pediatric patients with open physes, and as adjuvant therapy with other constructs.

- The surgical technique employed should make an effort to capture the involved fracture fragments when possible in an effort to limit the risk of redisplacement.

- K-wires should remain in place until the patient is nontender over the fracture, which often occurs between weeks 4 and 6 following surgery.

- Immobilization after surgery should immobilize only the necessary joints when possible

- and should be tailored to the specific patient and fracture pattern.
- Outcomes of CRPP for distal radius fractures are favorable when applied in the correct setting, taking into account patient-related characteristics and fracture.
- Common complications include loss of reduction, pin tract infection, pin migration, and skin irritation. Patients need to be warned accordingly for expectation regulation should these issues arise.

DISCLOSURES

M.B. Gottschalk receives research support from Stryker, Konica Minolta, and Arthrex. E.R. Wagner receives research support from Konica Minolta and Arthrex and is a consultant for Stryker.

REFERENCES

1. Chung KC, Spilson SV. The frequency and epidemiology of hand and forearm fractures in the United States. J Hand Surg Am 2001;26(5):908–15.
2. Nellans KW, Kowalski E, Chung KC. The epidemiology of distal radius fractures. Hand Clin 2012; 28(2):113–25.
3. Chung KC, Shauver MJ, Birkmeyer JD. Trends in the United States in the treatment of distal radial fractures in the elderly. J Bone Joint Surg Am 2009; 91(8):1868–73.
4. Lafontaine M, Hardy D, Delince P. Stability assessment of distal radius fractures. Injury 1989;20(4): 208–10.
5. Mackenney PJ, McQueen MM, Elton R. Prediction of instability in distal radial fractures. J Bone Joint Surg Am 2006;88(9):1944–51.
6. LaMartina J, Jawa A, Stucken C, et al. Predicting alignment after closed reduction and casting of distal radius fractures. J Hand Surg Am 2015; 40(5):934–9.
7. Santoshi JA, Chaware PN, Pakhare AP, et al. An anatomical study to demonstrate the proximity of kirschner wires to structures at risk in percutaneous pinning of distal radius fractures. J Hand Microsurg 2015;7(1):73–8.
8. Sengab A, Krijnen P, Schipper IB. Risk factors for fracture redisplacement after reduction and cast immobilization of displaced distal radius fractures in children: a meta-analysis. Eur J Trauma Emerg Surg 2020;46(4):789–800.
9. Shehovych A, Salar O, Meyer C, et al. Adult distal radius fractures classification systems: essential clinical knowledge or abstract memory testing? Ann R Coll Surg Engl 2016;98(8):525–31.
10. Diaz-Garcia RJ, Chung KC. The evolution of distal radius fracture management: a historical treatise. Hand Clin 2012;28(2):105–11.
11. Rayhack JM. The history and evolution of percutaneous pinning of displaced distal radius fractures. Orthop Clin North Am 1993;24(2):287–300.
12. Castaing J. Recent Fractures of the Lower Extremity of the Radius in Adults. Rev Chir Orthop Reparatrice Appar Mot 1964;50:581–696.
13. Docquier J, Soete P, Twahirwa J, et al. Kapandji's method of intrafocal nailing in Pouteau-Colles fractures. Acta Orthop Belg 1982;48(5):794–810.
14. Freising S, Walter B. Conservative and surgical treatment of radius fractures loco classico. Chirurgia 1983;54(11):742–8.
15. Kerboul B, Le Saout J, Lefevre C, et al. Comparative study of 3 therapeutic methods for Pouteau Colles' fracture. Apropos of 97 cases. J Chir (Paris) 1986; 123(6–7):428–34.
16. Willenegger H, Guggenbuhl A. Operative treatment of certain cases of distal radius fracture. Helv Chir Acta 1959;26(2):81–94.
17. Mah ET, Atkinson RN. Percutaneous Kirschner wire stabilisation following closed reduction of Colles' fractures. J Hand Surg Br 1992;17(1):55–62.
18. DePALMA AF. Comminuted fractures of the distal end of the radius treated by ulnar pinning. J Bone Joint Surg Am 1952;24 A(3):651–62.
19. Stein AH Jr, Katz SF. Stabilization of comminuted fractures of the distal inch of the radius: percutaneous pinning. Clin Orthop Relat Res 1975;(108): 174–81.
20. Kapandji A. [Internal fixation by double intrafocal plate. Functional treatment of non articular fractures of the lower end of the radius (author's transl)]. Ann Chir 1976;30(11–12):903–8.
21. Kapandji A. Intra-focal pinning of fractures of the distal end of the radius 10 years later. Ann Chir Main 1987;6(1):57–63.
22. Rayhack JM, Langworthy JN, Belsole RJ. Transulnar percutaneous pinning of displaced distal radial fractures: a preliminary report. J Orthop Trauma 1989; 3(2):107–14.
23. Vidyadharan A. A novel method of closed reduction and percutaneous pinning with six K-wires for intra-articular fractures of the distal radius. J Am Acad Orthop Surg Glob Res Rev 2020;4(6).
24. Koval KJ, Harrast JJ, Anglen JO, et al. Fractures of the distal part of the radius. The evolution of practice over time. Where's the evidence? J Bone Joint Surg Am 2008;90(9):1855–61.
25. Childs S, Mann T, Dahl J, et al. Differences in the treatment of distal radius fractures by hand fellowship trained surgeons: a study of ABOS candidate data. J Hand Surg Am 2017;42(2):e91–7.
26. Hinds RM, Capo JT, Kakar S, et al. Early complications following osteosynthesis of distal radius

fractures: a comparison of geriatric and nongeriatric cohorts. Geriatr Orthop Surg Rehabil 2017;8(1):30–3.

27. Bong MR, Egol KA, Leibman M, et al. A comparison of immediate postreduction splinting constructs for controlling initial displacement of fractures of the distal radius: a prospective randomized study of long-arm versus short-arm splinting. J Hand Surg Am 2006;31(5):766–70.

28. Gamba C, Fernandez FAM, Llavall MC, et al. Which immobilization is better for distal radius fracture? A prospective randomized trial. Int Orthop 2017; 41(9):1723–7.

29. Tumia N, Wardlaw D, Hallett J, et al. Aberdeen Colles' fracture brace as a treatment for Colles' fracture. A multicentre, prospective, randomised, controlled trial. J Bone Joint Surg Br 2003;85(1): 78–82.

30. Wahlstrom O. Treatment of Colles' fracture. A prospective comparison of three different positions of immobilization. Acta Orthop Scand 1982;53(2): 225–8.

31. Caruso G, Tonon F, Gildone A, et al. Below-elbow or above-elbow cast for conservative treatment of extra-articular distal radius fractures with dorsal displacement: a prospective randomized trial. J Orthop Surg Res 2019;14(1):477.

32. Rahman AM, Montero-Lopez N, Hinds RM, et al. Assessment of forearm rotational control using 4 upper extremity immobilization constructs. Hand (N Y). 2018;13(2):202–8.

33. Strickland J, Steichen J, Kleinman W, et al. Phalangeal fractures. Factors influenceing digital performance. Orthop Rev 1982;11:39–50.

34. Karantana A, Handoll HH, Sabouni A. Percutaneous pinning for treating distal radial fractures in adults. Cochrane Database Syst Rev 2020;2: CD006080.

35. Costa ML, Achten J, Parsons NR, et al. Percutaneous fixation with Kirschner wires versus volar locking plate fixation in adults with dorsally displaced fracture of distal radius: randomised controlled trial. BMJ 2014;349:g4807.

36. Costa ML, Achten J, Rangan A, et al. Percutaneous fixation with Kirschner wires versus volar locking-plate fixation in adults with dorsally displaced fracture of distal radius: five-year follow-up of a randomized controlled trial. Bone Joint J 2019;101-B(8): 978–83.

37. Goehre F, Otto W, Schwan S, et al. Comparison of palmar fixed-angle plate fixation with K-wire fixation of distal radius fractures (AO A2, A3, C1) in elderly patients. J Hand Surg Eur 2014;39(3):249–57.

38. Hollevoet N, Vanhoutie T, Vanhove W, et al. Percutaneous K-wire fixation versus palmar plating with locking screws for Colles' fractures. Acta Orthop Belg 2011;77(2):180–7.

39. Karantana A, Downing ND, Forward DP, et al. Surgical treatment of distal radial fractures with a volar locking plate versus conventional percutaneous methods: a randomized controlled trial. J Bone Joint Surg Am 2013;95(19):1737–44.

40. Marcheix PS, Dotzis A, Benko PE, et al. Extension fractures of the distal radius in patients older than 50: a prospective randomized study comparing fixation using mixed pins or a palmar fixed-angle plate. J Hand Surg Eur 2010;35(8):646–51.

41. McFadyen I, Field J, McCann P, et al. Should unstable extra-articular distal radial fractures be treated with fixed-angle volar-locked plates or percutaneous Kirschner wires? A prospective randomised controlled trial. Injury 2011;42(2):162–6.

42. Rozental TD, Blazar PE, Franko OI, et al. Functional outcomes for unstable distal radial fractures treated with open reduction and internal fixation or closed reduction and percutaneous fixation. A prospective randomized trial. J Bone Joint Surg Am 2009;91(8): 1837–46.

43. Chaudhry H, Kleinlugtenbelt YV, Mundi R, et al. Are volar locking plates superior to percutaneous K-wires for distal radius fractures? A Meta-analysis. Clin Orthop Relat Res 2015;473(9):3017–27.

44. Franchignoni F, Vercelli S, Giordano A, et al. Minimal clinically important difference of the disabilities of the arm, shoulder and hand outcome measure (DASH) and its shortened version (QuickDASH). J Orthop Sports Phys Ther 2014;44(1):30–9.

45. Dzaja I, MacDermid JC, Roth J, et al. Functional outcomes and cost estimation for extra-articular and simple intra-articular distal radius fractures treated with open reduction and internal fixation versus closed reduction and percutaneous Kirschner wire fixation. Can J Surg 2013;56(6):378–84.

46. Mathews AL, Chung KC. Management of complications of distal radius fractures. Hand Clin 2015;31(2): 205–15.

47. Liao Q, Skipper NC, Brown MJ, et al. Percutaneous pinning versus volar locking plate fixation for dorsally displaced distal radius fractures- reoperation rates over an eight year period. J Orthop 2018;15(2):471–4.

Plate Fixation of Distal Radius Fractures
What Type of Plate to Use and When?

Lili E. Schindelar, MD, MPH, Asif M. Ilyas, MD, MBA*

KEYWORDS

- Distal radius fracture • Volar plate • Dorsal plate • Bridge plate • Open reduction internal fixation

KEY POINTS

- Volar locking plates have broad fracture applicability, a reasonable soft tissue profile, and consistent outcomes.
- Dorsal locking plates provide the advantages of direct fracture exposure, stable fixation for dorsal shear fractures, and better access to dorsal die-punch fractures and fractures with significant dorsal bone loss requiring bone grafting.
- Bridge plates can span highly comminuted fractures and are left in situ until complete fracture healing, while possessing a lower complication profile than external fixators.
- Bridge plates are beneficial for the polytraumatized patient to aid in immediate weight bearing for transfers and rehabilitation.

With innovations in plating design and technique, plate fixation of distal radius fractures has seen increasing popularity. Advances in plate technology, such as locking constructs and variable angle screws, have led to its use in the majority of surgically treated fractures. Moreover, a number of plate fixation options are available to surgically manage distal radius fractures, including, volar, dorsal, and bridge plating. This article outlines the current concepts of plate fixation of distal radius fractures with the recent literature to better define indications for use.

The goal of distal radius fracture fixation is to obtain anatomic reduction and stable fixation for early mobilization and preserved functionality. A recent meta-analysis showed that plate fixation provides the best outcomes in terms of early functional recovery and lower complication rates, as compared with external fixation, intramedullary nailing, K-wires, or casting.[1] There are many plating techniques and designs to manage distal radius fractures; however, there is no consensus in the literature as to which is the most advantageous. Thus, the type of plate used should be dictated by fracture characteristics, patient factors, and surgeon experience.

VOLAR PLATING

Fixation of a distal radius fracture with a volar buttress plate is a well-recognized fixation strategy for volar shear fractures that has been espoused for several decades through traditional AO training.[2] However, aside from these "volar (shear) Barton" fractures, most distal radius fractures indicated for surgical repair through the end of the twentieth century had been treated with either pins and plaster, percutaneous pinning and casting, external fixation, or dorsal buttress plate fixation.[3] But over the past 20 plus years, volar locking plate fixation has become the fixation treatment of choice.[4] Popularized by Orbay, the volar locking plate design allowed for volar plate fixation of dorsally angulated fractures through

The Rothman Orthopaedic Institute, Thomas Jefferson University, Rothman Institute, 925 Chestnut Street, 5th Floor, Philadelphia, PA 19107, USA
* Corresponding author. Rothman Institute, 925 Chestnut Street, 5th Floor, Philadelphia, PA 19107.
E-mail address: asif.ilyas@rothmanortho.com

Hand Clin 37 (2021) 259–266
https://doi.org/10.1016/j.hcl.2021.02.008

hand.theclinics.com

its fixed angle construct, thereby avoiding the soft tissue problems common with dorsal plate fixation.[5,6] Subsequently, the volar locking plate technique has continued to grow in popularity and use for several reasons. First, volar locking plates have broad fracture applicability, because they can be applied for nearly all fractures patterns, including AO types A, B, and C patterns, with the primary contraindication being radiocarpal fracture dislocations with a radial styloid avulsion (AO type B1), and dorsal shear patterns (AO type B2), aka "dorsal Barton" fractures. Second, the surgical technique has a relatively low complication incidence, with the low-profile plate under a robust soft tissue envelope, and a low associated soft tissue injury rate, such as tendon ruptures.[7,8] Last, volar locking plates have produced consistently good surgical outcomes.[9–14]

There are many types of volar plates that are available to surgically manage distal radius fractures. Current plate designs include nonlocking, locking fixed angle, and locking variable angle plates. Nonlocking volar plates remain applicable for "volar (shear) Barton" fracture patterns. However, locking technology has revolutionized periarticular fracture fixations, such as distal radius fractures, by allowing the plate and screws to act as a single unit that does not rely on the integrity of the subchondral bone for a stable construct, while also avoiding bicortical periarticular fixation.[15] In addition, biomechanical studies have shown that locked plates can increase fracture construct strength by more than 4 times compared with its nonlocking counterparts.[16,17] Locked plate designs also allow stresses to be transmitted to the subchondral bone, rather than the weakened bone at the fracture site, which creates increased rigidity and a stable construct for potentially early mobilization.[16] Furthermore, locked plates can be positioned along the volar cortex and have the potential to control dorsally displaced fractures from distal screws extending below the subchondral surface.[18] The first locked volar plate designed was a fixed angle construct, which has a predetermined volar tilt and radial inclination designed into the plate, with the distal locking screws also at a predetermined angle.[6] In contrast, newer constructs offer a variable angle design of the distal screws, with 30° to 40° of variability between the locking screw and the plate.[19] This construction allows the surgeon to determine the direction of the distal subchondral screws, offering the potential to place a screw into specific fracture fragments for increased fixation (**Fig. 1**).[16] In addition, with increased understanding of the effects of subchondral screws with potential soft tissue irritation or cut out, newer distal locking

constructs are now available, including smooth pegs, with the theoretic advantage of less extensor tendon irritation while still providing subchondral support.[19] Biomechanical studies have shown smooth pegs to be significantly weaker than screws in the distal fragment, but the difference may not be clinically signficant.[20,21] However, another clinical study found no difference in stability between the two.[22]

The recent literature on outcomes after volar locking plate fixation of distal radius fractures has shown overall superior results as compared with other fixation techniques. Fu and colleagues[11] performed a meta-analysis of randomized controlled trials comparing volar locking plates with external fixation for distal radius fractures and found superior outcomes in terms of functional outcome scores, range of motion, and complications in the volar plating group. Other meta-analyses have also reported better functional outcomes after volar locking plates as compared with external fixators, as well as better radiographic outcomes in the plating group.[12,23] When compared with dorsal plates, volar locking plates have been found to have comparable functional outcomes.[24,25] However, 1 prospective cohort study demonstrated better range of motion and grip strength with volar plating as compared with dorsal plates.[26] Multiple randomized controlled trials have shown better functional outcomes after volar locked plating of distal radius fractures as compared with nonoperative treatment.[10,27] Although it is now common practice to treat younger patients with a distal radius fracture with volar plating over nonoperative treatment, the elderly population have had more inconsistent results regarding these 2 treatments.[28–30] However, newer randomized controlled trials have demonstrated superior and comparable functional outcomes following volar locked plating versus nonoperative treatment in the elderly, with comparable complication rates.[31–33]

In a recent analysis between variable angle versus fixed angle volar locking plates, fixed angle plates were found to have significantly more complications.[34] The majority of complications with fixed angle plates were related to prominent or poorly positioned hardware.[34] Fixed angle plates are designed to be placed in a specific location to optimize subchondral support along the articular surface, and have a limited range to how far they can be positioned distally to avoid intra-articular screw placement. In contrast, another prospective study of unstable distal radius fractures treated with variable angle volar plates produced acceptable reduction in all patients and excellent clinical outcomes at the 1-year follow-

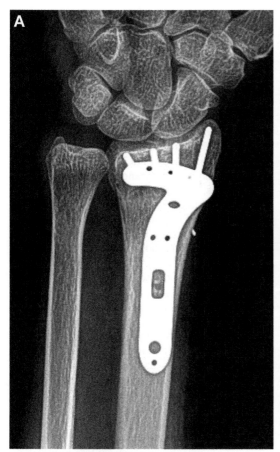
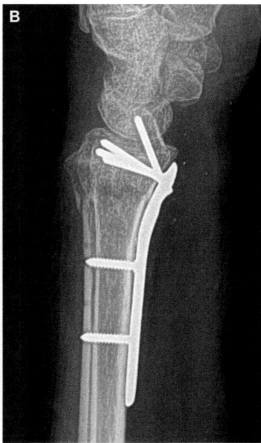

Fig. 1. (*A*) AP and (*B*) lateral radiograph of a distal radius fracture treated with a volar locking variable-angle plate with distal smooth pegs (Globus, Audubon, PA). (*Courtesy of* Asif M. Ilyas, MD, MBA, FACS; with permission.)

up.[35] The major disadvantage of variable angle designs is their cost, which can be up to 10 times the cost of standard plate designs.[16]

Looking more closely at associated complications with locked volar plating, a systematic review by Alter and colleagues[7] found an overall complication rate of 15%, with nerve dysfunction to be the most common complication, occurring in about 5% of cases, followed by tendon dysfunction in about 3% of cases. Similarly, Thorninger and colleagues[36] found that, upon review of more than 500 distal radius fracture cases, carpal tunnel syndrome and tendon injuries were also the most common complications. Other common complications associated with volar locked plates relate to hardware placement. For example, volar plate prominence beyond the watershed line can cause flexor tendon injury, and dorsal penetration of screws or pegs can lead to extensor tendon injury. Moreover, the incidence of removal for symptomatic hardware has been reported at 7%.[18] Therefore, careful positioning of volar plates to avoid volar prominence and intra-articular

screw penetration, as well as appropriate selection of screw length to reduce irritation of extensor tendons, can decrease avoidable complications in these constructs.

DORSAL PLATING

Before volar locked plates, nonlocking dorsal plates were commonly used for the fixation of dorsally comminuted fractures of the distal radius. The dorsal approach to the distal radius is attractive in that it provides direct visualization and reduction of the fracture site, whereas a volar approach provides a relatively indirect reduction. The dorsal plate can also act as a buttress against dorsal collapse, creating a biomechanically superior construct in some fracture patterns.[37] However, the proximity of the plates to the extensor tendons lends to the historically high rate of complications for this technique. However, like volar plates, newer dorsal plate designs have also incorporated locking technology and a lower and more anatomic profile in an effort to decrease extensor tendon irritation. There are 2 general types of dorsal plate designs, namely, buttress type plates and column plates.[16] Buttress type plates have a T-type design and are designed to broadly resist dorsal displacement or collapse, whereas column plates are meant to anatomically repair the radial and ulnar columns of the dorsal distal radius (**Fig. 2**).[16] The indications for dorsal plating include dorsal (shear) Barton fractures, dorsal die-punch fractures, fractures with significant dorsal comminution potentially requiring bone grafting, and correction of dorsal malunions.[24]

Recent evidence comparing low-profile dorsal locked plates with the historically thicker dorsal nonlocking pi plates showed more complications and a higher revision rate with pi plates.[38] In contrast, newer dorsal locking plates have demonstrated improved complication rates and functional outcomes.[24,25,39–42] Overall, complications are typically related to extensor tendon irritation, but dorsal plates have also been related to neurologic complications as with volar plates.[25,41,42] Similarly, functional and radiographic outcomes after dorsal locked plating have been acceptable and comparable to volar locked plating.[24,25,39,41]

BRIDGE PLATING

Wrist-spanning dorsal bridge plates provide an alternative fixation option for distal radius fractures. Dorsal bridge plating can be considered analogous to an internal external fixator. Indications for the use of bridge plating include the management of distal radius fractures with extensive articular comminution, dorsal (shear) Barton fractures, and fractures with radial meta-diaphyseal comminution.[43] Additional indications include the neutralization of simple and complex radiocarpal dislocations, or the neutralization of distal radius fractures to allow immediate weight-bearing in patients who are "functional quadrupeds," or patients who require all their limbs to weight bear on walkers and crutches.[44]

In terms of design rationale, similar to external fixation, bridge plating consists of closed or limited open reduction of the fracture followed by spanning wrist internal fixation with ligamentotaxis.[45] Unlike external fixation, the implant is entirely deep to the skin, thereby avoiding pin track complications and with the added advantage of keeping the hardware in as long as necessary. Also unlike external fixation, the dorsal position of the plate provides for a buttress effect for dorsally

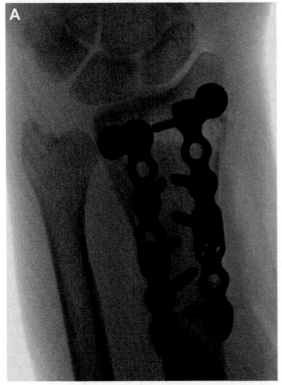
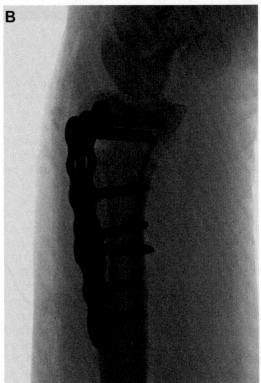

Fig. 2. (*A*) AP and (*B*) lateral radiographs of a distal radius fracture treated with dorsal column plating (Globus, Audubon, PA). (*Courtesy of* Asif M. Ilyas, MD, MBA, FACS; with permission.)

unstable fracture patterns (**Fig. 3**). However, because the hardware is placed deep, a return to the operating room for staged removal of hardware is necessary.

An advantage of bridge plates is that they can be left in place for much longer than external fixation devices. However, plates are typically left in situ for 2 to 3 months, until there is adequate fracture healing before they are removed, whereas external fixators must be removed sooner owing to the higher risk of pin site irritation or infections. Additionally, bridge plates offer unrestricted use of the hand and immediate weight bearing through the wrist. This offers benefits for the polytrauma patient who may require early mobilization with assistive devices for lower extremity injuries.

The major disadvantage is the necessity of a second surgery for plate removal. There are also concerns for postoperative stiffness and decreased strength because the plate spans the wrist joint for an extended period of immobilization.[45–47]

Despite these disadvantages, the literature on outcomes after bridge plating of distal radius fractures demonstrates acceptable functionality and low complication rates. A recent meta-analysis examining outcomes of bridge plating found lower complication rates as compared with external fixation.[46] Complications of external fixation of distal radius fractures have typically been related to infection, and rates in the literature range from 23% to 62%.[46–48] A recent study comparing the complication rates of bridge plating to external fixation showed a significantly lower infection rate in bridge plating (2% vs 10%), as well as a lower rate of complex regional pain syndrome (1% vs 4%).[49]

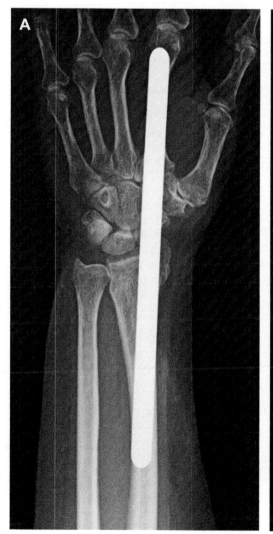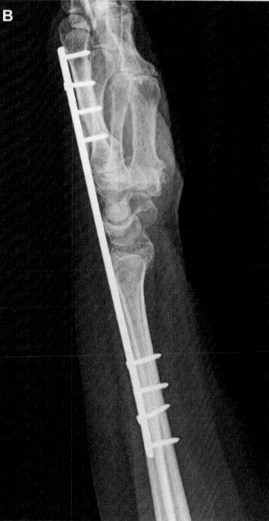

Fig. 3. (*A*) AP and (*B*) lateral radiographs of a distal radius fracture treated with a dorsal bridge plate (Globus, Audubon, PA). (*Courtesy of* Asif M. Ilyas, MD, MBA, FACS; with permission.)

Other data show complication rates after bridge plating to range from 1.6% to 12%, which are consistently lower than rates for external fixation.[46,47] Recent studies have found functional and radiographic outcomes to be comparable in bridge plating versus volar plating of distal radius fractures.[46] Range of motion was also shown to return to functional levels after plate removal in multiple studies.[46,47] Dorsal bridge plating may be a viable option for certain fracture patterns or patient characteristics that may otherwise be unstable with a periarticular plate.

SUMMARY

The treatment of distal radius fractures with plating aims to create a stable construct with anatomic reduction and early return to function. There are many options for the approach, the type of plate, and the method of reduction that can be used to reach this goal. Innovations in plate design, especially the volar plate, have led to excellent functional outcomes with low complication rates. Similarly, the dorsal plate is making advances with a slimmer profile and lower complication rate than historical nonlocking designs. Most recently, the bridge plate has emerged as a promising alternative to external fixation that reduces the issues of infection with pin sites. There is no panacea for plating all distal radius fractures; instead, the type of plate used should depend on the experience of the surgeon, the type of fracture, and patient characteristics.

CLINICS CARE POINTS

- Volar locking plates have broad fracture applicability, a reasonable soft tissue profile, and consistent outcomes.

- Dorsal locking plates provide the advantages of direct fracture exposure, stable fixation for dorsal shear fractures, and better access to dorsal die-punch fractures and fractures with significant dorsal bone loss requiring bone grafting.

- Bridge plates can span highly comminuted fractures and are left in situ until complete fracture healing, while possessing a lower complication profile than external fixators.

- Bridge plates are beneficial for the polytraumatized patient to aid in immediate weight bearing for transfers and rehabilitation.

DISCLOSURE

Dr L.E. Schindelar has nothing to disclose. Dr A.M. Ilyas is a consultant for Acumed, AxoGen and Globus Medical; is a paid presenter or speaker for DePuy; receives IP royalties from Globus Medical; and is a board or committee member for the PA Ortho Society.

REFERENCES

1. Vannabouathong C, Hussain N, Guerra-Farfan E, et al. Interventions for distal radius fractures: a network meta-analysis of randomized trials. J Am Acad Orthop Surg 2019;27(13):e596–605.
2. Fernández DL. Fractures of the distal radius: operative treatment. Instr Course Lect 1993;42:73–88.
3. Ilyas AM, Jupiter JB. Distal radius fractures—classification of treatment and indications for surgery. Hand Clin 2010;26(1):37–42.
4. Koval KJ, Harrast JJ, Anglen JO, et al. Fractures of the distal part of the radius. The evolution of practice over time. Where's the evidence? J Bone Joint Surg Am 2008;90(9):1855–61.
5. Orbay JL, Fernandez DL. Volar fixation for dorsally displaced fractures of the distal radius: a preliminary report. J Hand Surg 2002;27(2):205–15.
6. Orbay JL. The treatment of unstable distal radius fractures with volar fixation. Hand Surg 2000; 05(02):103–12.
7. Alter TH, Sandrowski K, Gallant G, et al. Complications of volar plating of distal radius fractures: a systematic review. J Wrist Surg 2019;08(03):255–62.
8. Alter TH, Ilyas AM. Complications associated with volar locking plate fixation of distal radial fractures. JBJS Rev 2018;6(10):e7.
9. Yu X, Yu Y, Shao X, et al. Volar locking plate versus external fixation with optional additional K-wire for treatment of AO type C2/C3 fractures: a retrospective comparative study. J Orthop Surg 2019;14(1): 271.
10. Mulders MAM, Walenkamp MMJ, van Dieren S, et al. Volar plate fixation versus plaster immobilization in acceptably reduced extra-articular distal radial fractures: a multicenter randomized controlled trial. J Bone Joint Surg Am 2019;101(9):787–96.
11. Fu Q, Zhu L, Yang P, et al. Volar locking plate versus external fixation for distal radius fractures: a meta-analysis of randomized controlled trials. Indian J Orthop 2018;52(6):602.
12. Wang J, Lu Y, Cui Y, et al. Is volar locking plate superior to external fixation for distal radius fractures? A comprehensive meta-analysis. Acta Orthop Traumatol Turc 2018;52(5):334–42.
13. Quadlbauer S, Pezzei Ch, Jurkowitsch J, et al. Functional and radiological outcome of distal radius fractures stabilized by volar-locking plate with a

minimum follow-up of 1 year. Arch Orthop Trauma Surg 2020. https://doi.org/10.1007/s00402-020-03411-9.

14. Roh YH, Lee BK, Baek JR, et al. A randomized comparison of volar plate and external fixation for intraarticular distal radius fractures. J Hand Surg 2015; 40(1):34–41.

15. Joglekar S, Ilyas A. The role of locking technology in the upper extremity. J Hand Microsurg 2016;01(02): 82–91.

16. Loisel F, Kielwasser H, Faivre G, et al. Treatment of distal radius fractures with locking plates: an update. Eur J Orthop Surg Traumatol 2018;28(8): 1537–42.

17. Obert L, Rey P-B, Uhring J, et al. Fixation of distal radius fractures in adults: a review. Orthop Traumatol Surg Res 2013;99(2):216–34.

18. Wilson J, Viner JJ, Johal KS, et al. Volar locking plate fixations for displaced distal radius fractures: an evaluation of complications and radiographic outcomes. Hand (N Y) 2018;13(4):466–72.

19. Park JH, Hagopian J, Ilyas AM. Variable-angle locking screw volar plating of distal radius fractures. Hand Clin 2010;26(3):373–80.

20. Martineau PA, Waitayawinyu T, Malone KJ, et al. Volar plating of AO C3 distal radius fractures: biomechanical evaluation of locking screw and locking smooth peg configurations. J Hand Surg 2008; 33(6):827–34.

21. Weninger P, Dall'Ara E, Leixnering M, et al. Volar fixed-angle plating of extra-articular distal radius fractures—a biomechanical analysis comparing threaded screws and smooth pegs. J Trauma 2010;69(5):E46–55.

22. Boretto JG, Pacher N, Giunta D, et al. Comparative clinical study of locking screws versus smooth locking pegs in volar plating of distal radius fractures. J Hand Surg Eur 2014;39(7):755–60.

23. Gouk CJC, Bindra RR, Tarrant DJ, et al. Volar locking plate fixation versus external fixation of distal radius fractures: a meta-analysis. J Hand Surg Eur 2018; 43(9):954–60.

24. Abe Y, Tokunaga S, Moriya T. Management of intraarticular distal radius fractures: volar or dorsal locking plate—which has fewer complications? Hand (N Y) 2017;12(6):561–7.

25. Kumar S, Khan AN, Sonanis SV. Radiographic and functional evaluation of low profile dorsal versus volar plating for distal radius fractures. J Orthop 2016;13(4):376–82.

26. Jakubietz MG, Gruenert JG, Jakubietz RG. Palmar and dorsal fixed-angle plates in AO C-type fractures of the distal radius: is there an advantage of palmar plates in the long term? J Orthop Surg 2012;7(1):8.

27. Sharma H, Khare GN, Singh S, et al. Outcomes and complications of fractures of distal radius (AO type B and C): volar plating versus nonoperative treatment. J Orthop Sci 2014;19(4):537–44.

28. Diaz-Garcia RJ, Oda T, Shauver MJ, et al. A systematic review of outcomes and complications of treating unstable distal radius fractures in the elderly. J Hand Surg 2011;36(5):824–35.e2.

29. Chen Y, Chen X, Li Z, et al. Safety and efficacy of operative versus nonsurgical management of distal radius fractures in elderly patients: a systematic review and meta-analysis. J Hand Surg 2016;41(3): 404–13.

30. Arora R, Gabl M, Gschwentner M, et al. A comparative study of clinical and radiologic outcomes of unstable Colles type distal radius fractures in patients older than 70 years: nonoperative treatment versus volar locking plating. J Orthop Trauma 2009;23(4):237–42.

31. Arora R, Lutz M, Deml C, et al. A prospective randomized trial comparing nonoperative treatment with volar locking plate fixation for displaced and unstable distal radial fractures in patients sixty-five years of age and older. J Bone Joint Surg Am 2011;93(23):2146–53.

32. Saving J, Severin Wahlgren S, Olsson K, et al. Nonoperative treatment compared with volar locking plate fixation for dorsally displaced distal radial fractures in the elderly: a randomized controlled trial. J Bone Joint Surg Am 2019;101(11):961–9.

33. Martinez-Mendez D, Lizaur-Utrilla A, de-Juan-Herrero J. Intra-articular distal radius fractures in elderly patients: a randomized prospective study of casting versus volar plating. J Hand Surg Eur 2018;43(2):142–7.

34. Mehrzad R, Kim DC. Complication rate comparing variable angle distal locking plate to fixed angle plate fixation of distal radius fractures. Ann Plast Surg 2016;77(6):623–5.

35. Fowler JR, Ilyas AM. Prospective evaluation of distal radius fractures treated with variable-angle volar locking plates. J Hand Surg 2013;38(11): 2198–203.

36. Thorninger R, Madsen ML, Wæver D, et al. Complications of volar locking plating of distal radius fractures in 576 patients with 3.2 years follow-up. Injury 2017;48(6):1104–9.

37. Leixnering M, Rosenauer R, Pezzei Ch, et al. Indications, surgical approach, reduction, and stabilization techniques of distal radius fractures. Arch Orthop Trauma Surg 2020. https://doi.org/10.1007/s00402-020-03365-y.

38. Rozental TD, Beredjiklian PK, Bozentka DJ. Functional outcome and complications following two types of dorsal plating for unstable fractures of the distal part of the radius. J Bone Joint Surg Am 2003;85(10):1956–60.

39. Matzon JL, Kenniston J, Beredjiklian PK. Hardware-related complications after dorsal plating for displaced distal radius fractures. Orthopedics 2014; 37(11):e978–82.

40. Wei J, Yang T-B, Luo W, et al. Complications following dorsal versus volar plate fixation of distal radius fracture: a meta-analysis. J Int Med Res 2013;41(2):265–75.

41. Disseldorp DJG, Hannemann PFW, Poeze M, et al. Dorsal or volar plate fixation of the distal radius: does the complication rate help us to choose? J Wrist Surg 2016;05(03):202–10.

42. Yu YR, Makhni MC, Tabrizi S, et al. Complications of low-profile dorsal versus volar locking plates in the distal radius: a comparative study. J Hand Surg 2011;36(7):1135–41.

43. Burke EF, Singer RM. Treatment of comminuted distal radius with the use of an internal distraction plate. Tech Hand Up Extrem Surg 1998;2(4):248–52.

44. Tinsley BA, Ilyas AM. Distal radius fractures in a functional quadruped. Hand Clin 2018;34(1): 113–20.

45. Dodds SD, Save AV, Yacob A. Dorsal spanning plate fixation for distal radius fractures. Tech Hand Up Extrem Surg 2013;17(4):192–8.

46. Perlus R, Doyon J, Henry P. The use of dorsal distraction plating for severely comminuted distal radius fractures: a review and comparison to volar plate fixation. Injury 2019;50:S50–5.

47. Lauder A, Agnew S, Bakri K, et al. Functional outcomes following bridge plate fixation for distal radius fractures. J Hand Surg 2015;40(8): 1554–62.

48. Vakhshori V, Alluri RK, Stevanovic M, et al. Review of internal radiocarpal distraction plating for distal radius fracture fixation. Hand (N Y) 2020;15(1): 116–24.

49. Wang WL, Ilyas AM. Dorsal bridge plating versus external fixation for distal radius fractures. J Wrist Surg 2020;09(02):177–84.

Strategies for Specific Reduction in High-Energy Distal Radius Fractures

Nicholas Pulos, MD, Alexander Y. Shin, MD*

KEYWORDS

- Distal radius fracture • Fragment-specific fixation • Distal radioulnar joint • Open reduction
- Internal fixation

KEY POINTS

- High-energy distal radius fractures result in predictable fragmentation of the subchondral bone and articular cartilage.
- Anatomic reduction requires visualization of the articular surface though multiple incisions or arthroscopy.
- Low-profile plating systems, designed specifically for each fragment type, allows for stable fixation of individual fragments.
- Distraction bridge plating and external fixation can be used to augment unstable distal radius fractures after anatomic reduction and small fragment fixation and should be considered only when necessary.

INTRODUCTION

The incidence of distal radius fractures demonstrates a bimodal distribution with low-energy fractures seen in osteoporotic elderly patients and high-energy fractures seen in a younger patients.[1] In addition to osseous injuries, high-energy distal radius fractures are often associated with injuries to skin, tendons, ligaments, and neurovascular structures.[2] Radiocarpal ligament attachments and trabecular ultrastructure of bone within the distal radius and lead to consistent fracture patterns demonstrated even among elderly patients with low-energy falls.[3–5] The ideal treatment restores articular congruity and carpal alignment. Our algorithm for surgical treatment of high-energy distal radius fractures using fragment-specific principles is presented.

CLASSIFICATION

Classification of distal radius fractures ranges from simple eponyms (ie, Colles fracture) to complex systems oriented toward research (ie, AO/OTA).[6] Several investigators have recognized common and consistent fracture patterns in their classification schemes including Melone,[7] Frykman,[8] and Jupiter and Fernandez.[9] A thorough knowledge of predictable patterns of fragmentation and the interpretation of injury radiographs is essential when taking care of these patients.[10]

Mandziak and colleagues[3] proposed articular fractures of the distal radius are more likely to occur between ligament attachments. Thus, the extrinsic ligaments of the wrist provide a roadmap of the location of fracture patterns. Although a high-energy distal radius fracture can result in an infinite combination of fracture fragments, there are 5 typical articular fragments that have the potential to be reduced and secured to a stable metadiaphyseal segment. These are the *volar ulnar corner* (also called the volar ulnar rim) and *dorsal ulnar corner*, which together form the sigmoid notch and portion of the lunate fossa; the *dorsal wall* and *free-intra-articular fragment*, which with

200 1st Street Southwest, Rochester, MN 55905, USA
* Corresponding author.
E-mail address: Shin.Alexander@mayo.edu
Twitter: @NickPulosMD (N.P.)

Hand Clin 37 (2021) 267–278
https://doi.org/10.1016/j.hcl.2021.02.009

the volar ulnar corner and dorsal ulnar corner fragments make up the lunate fossa; and the *radial styloid fragment*, which contains most of the scaphoid fossa (**Fig. 1**).

RADIOGRAPHIC EVALUATION

Initial radiographs include posterior-anterior (PA), oblique and lateral radiographs of the fracture before fracture reduction and demonstrate the tendency of the fracture to settle due to deforming forces.[11] Combining initial radiographs with traction films can reveal small, intra-articular fracture fragments that may be difficult to identify after closed reduction and splinting is performed (**Fig. 2**).

Common radiographic parameters used to describe distal radius displacement, such as volar tilt, radial height, and radial inclination, are useful for both extra-articular and intra-articular distal radius fractures. In high-energy distal radius fractures, 2 additional markers of displacement are beneficial. The teardrop angle represents the displacement of the volar ulnar corner. The normal teardrop angle is 70°, with lesser values indicating extension of the of the volar ulnar fragment. A widened anteroposterior distance of the distal radius represents articular incongruity between the dorsal and volar ulnar fragment, potentially

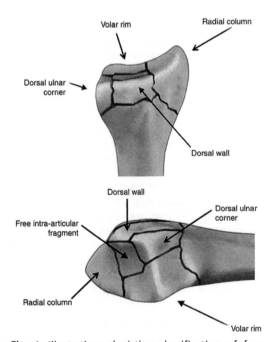

Fig. 1. Illustrations depicting classification of fragments that my result from a high-energy distal radius fracture. DUC, dorsal ulnar corner; DW, dorsal wall; RC, radial column; VUC, volar ulnar corner. (*Courtesy* Rhee PC, et al. J Am Acad Orthop Surg., 2017)

at the sigmoid notch. The average distance between the dorsal rim and volar rim is 17.8° in women and 20.4° in men and is roughly approximated by the width of the lunate on lateral radiographs.[10,12]

Computed tomography (CT) is not routinely necessary in the treatment of distal radius fractures but is helpful in high-energy fractures with intra-articular comminution to characterize the fracture, diagnose associated carpal injuries and develop a preoperative surgical plan.[13] Optimally, CT is obtained after closed reduction and immobilization is completed to place fragments in near normal positions that aid in identifying specific fragments (**Fig. 3**).

GENERAL CONSIDERATIONS

Before surgery in patients with high-energy distal radius fractures, the surgeon must take into account several patient-specific factors including age, comorbidities, associated injuries, and ambulatory status. For example, in polytrauma patients, the need for upper extremity weight bearing may lead the surgeon to augment fragment-specific fixation with a bridge plate or external fixator to allow for earlier weight bearing. Shared decision-making among elderly patients, patients with multiple comorbidities, their caregivers, and the surgeon may lead to nonoperative treatment in fractures that would otherwise benefit from open reduction and internal fixation.[14]

The timing of surgery may be outside the surgeon's control and depends at least partially on patient presentation, surgeon preference, and referral patterns. With highly comminuted distal radius fractures in particular, patients may be referred to several providers before ultimately presenting to a surgeon who specializes in treating these injuries. Fortunately, surgical delay does not appear to affect the ultimate outcome for the patient so long as the fracture is closed and not associated with nerve compression, compartment syndrome, or any other emergent surgical issues.[15] Early surgical treatment (<3 days) has the benefit of less distorted anatomy, less soft tissue swelling and scaring for the surgeon, and quicker recovery for the patient. Delaying surgery (>7 days) allows for soft tissue swelling, which can be impressive in high-energy distal radius fractures, to subside and more time for preoperative counseling of the patient regarding their upcoming surgery and impending convalescence. Depending on the patient and fracture, healing may start to occur by 3 weeks and delay beyond this point essentially turns the case into a malunion repair requiring corrective osteotomies.

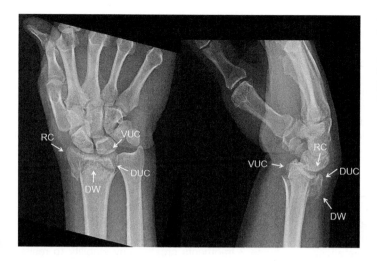

Fig. 2. PA and lateral radiographs with identifiable fracture fragments in a distal radius fracture with intra-articular comminution. DUC, dorsal ulnar corner; DW, dorsal wall; RC, radial column; VUC, volar ulnar corner.

Preoperative counseling has been shown to decrease the use of narcotic medication following upper extremity surgery.[16] The use of regional anesthesia with monitored anesthesia care is now common for these injuries. Long-acting anesthetic through the use of catheters or liposomal bupivacaine can provide sufficient relief that more than a quarter of patients require no opioid medications after surgery. Tylenol and nonsteroidal anti-inflammatory medications are encouraged, as well as ice, elevation, and edema control measures. Postoperative pain management, aggressive range of motion, and edema control are imperative to successful outcomes.

APPROACH TO TREATMENT

An algorithmic approach to high-energy distal radius fractures ensures that the complexity of the injury does not overwhelm the analytical process and prevents jumping of steps. It enables the optimal stepwise approach in restoring the articular surfaces of comminuted distal radius fractures. Restoration of radial height, radial inclination, and volar tilt with no more than 2 mm of articular incongruity remain the goals of surgical treatment. After application of appropriate fixation, a stable construct is created to prevent fracture displacement, allowing for early range of motion and ultimately leads to successful union and

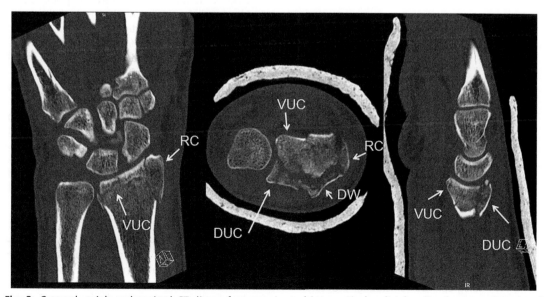

Fig. 3. Coronal, axial, and sagittal CT slices of a comminuted intra-articular distal radius fracture after closed reduction and splinting.

functional outcomes. The column model, which organizes the distal radius into an intermediate column, radial column, and pedestal and an additional column for the ulna, is the basis of our algorithm.[17] (**Fig. 4**)

Application of a fragment-specific approach uses multiple incisions that are strategically placed to address the major fragments of the distal radius fracture. Specially designed plates for specific fragments are applied.

Intermediate Column

The intermediate column contains the volar ulnar corner, dorsal ulnar corner, dorsal wall, and free intra-articular fragments. This column includes both the radiocarpal articulation (the lunate fossa) and the radioulnar articulation (sigmoid notch). Hara and colleagues[18] demonstrated that 35% of load transmission at the wrist occurs through the lunate facet. The restoration of the intermediate column allows for flexion/extension as well as pronotation/supination of the wrist and may arguably be the most critical column to anatomically reconstruct. To prevent a summative malreduction phenomenon, in which poor reduction of one fragment leads to subsequent poorer reduction of a subsequent fragment, it is essential to commence reduction with the most critical fragment, the volar ulnar corner.

The *volar ulnar corner fragment* is an attachment site for the short radiolunate ligament and the volar distal radioulnar ligament. Failure to adequately reduce and stabilize the volar ulnar corner

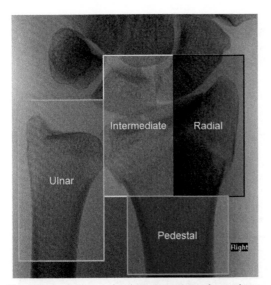

Fig. 4. PA radiograph demonstrating the column model of the distal radius and ulna. (*Adapted from* Rhee PC, et al. J Am Acad Orthop Surg., 2017.)

fragment can result in palmar displacement of the carpus, as seen with a volar Barton fracture. The volar ulnar corner has been identified as the most critical fragment.

The *dorsal ulnar corner fragment* is an attachment site for the dorsal radioulnar ligament and with the volar rim forms the sigmoid notch. Its only ligamentous attachment is to the distal ulna. Therefore, indirect reduction techniques and ligamentotaxis as performed when applying a bridge plate or external fixator are ineffective in achieving an anatomic reduction of this fragment. Distal traction results in further displacement and rotation of the dorsal ulnar fragment. The dorsal wall serves as an attachment site for the dorsal radiocarpal ligament. Together with the dorsal ulnar corner, these 2 fragments create bony stability to resist dorsal subluxation of the carpus.

Free intra-articular fragments contain variable amounts of the lunate and scaphoid facets. These fragments are most commonly impacted (proximally displaced) and with the fractures of the volar ulnar corner, dorsal ulnar corner and dorsal wall result in axial instability of the carpus and distal radius. Similar to the dorsal ulnar corner, free intra-articular fragments have no ligamentous attachment to the carpus, making anatomic reduction difficult with indirect techniques. These free intra-articular fragments often require subchondral bone grafting to provide stability.

Radial Column

The radial column contains the *radial styloid fragment,* which serves as the insertion site for the brachioradialis tendon and the radioscaphocapitate and long radiolunate ligaments. The radial column contains a radiocarpal articulation at the sigmoid notch, through which 50% of the axial load of the wrist is passed.[18] The radial column resists radial carpal translation as a bony buttress, but also prevents ulnar translation of the carpus through the radioscaphocapitate ligament. Although the main fracture line often runs in the sagittal plane through the interfossal ridge between the scaphoid and lunate facets, occasionally the radial column is comminuted with a split in the coronal plane through the scaphoid facet. This can be identified on radiographs as a double radial shadow or more definitively on preoperative CT imaging.

Pedestal

The *pedestal* is the metadiaphyseal radius on which the intermediate and radial column rest. This is the stable component and the base of any fracture fixation construct. With high-energy distal radius fractures, this segment may be comminuted with variable amounts of bone loss in open injuries.

Ulnar Column

The ulnar column consists of the distal ulna and triangular fibrocartilage complex (TFCC) through which 15% of the axial load through the wrist is transmitted.[18] The volar and dorsal distal radioulnar ligaments originating from the intermediate column insert on the ulnar column through superficial and deep fibers to the ulnar styloid and fovea, respectively. These ligamentous attachments are an essential component of forearm stability, permitting pronosupination through the distal radioulnar joint. The final operative consideration is stability of the distal radial ulnar joint (DRUJ) (**Fig. 5**).

SURGICAL APPROACHES AND REDUCTION TECHNIQUES
Intermediate Column

Through a volar approach over the flexor carpi radialis (FCR) tendon, also known as an FCR approach, the volar ulnar corner fragment may be difficult to visualize. By making an incision ulnar to the FCR, the tendon may be retracted

radially, allowing better access to the volar ulnar corner of the distal radius (**Fig. 6**). In some cases, radial retraction of the digital flexors may even be required to improve visualization. The pronator quadratus is elevated from radial to ulnar, and the distal attachment is carefully elevated ensuring the volar carpal ligaments are not divided. We routinely release the brachioradialis tendon to neutralize its deforming force on the radial styloid. Care should be taken to ensure that the volar ulnar corner fragment is well visualized with the pronator retracted. An angled Homan retractor placed just proximal to the DRUJ can help in this task.

Once the volar ulnar corner is visualized, a lobster claw is placed on the radial shaft and traction is applied to the hand to distract and disimpact the fracture. This may require some protonation or supination as well. The fracture site is debrided with a #15 blade, curette, and/or rongeur, and irrigated to remove any fracture hematoma and nonviable bony fragments. Reduction of the volar ulnar corner is performed under direct visualization using the proximal fracture line exiting out the volar ulnar cortex of the radius as guide. Occasionally a freer elevator is needed to lever out the volar ulnar corner fragment, or a dental pick needed to

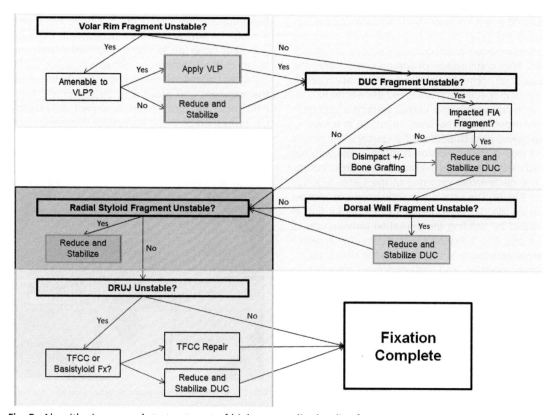

Fig. 5. Algorithmic approach to treatment of high-energy distal radius fractures.

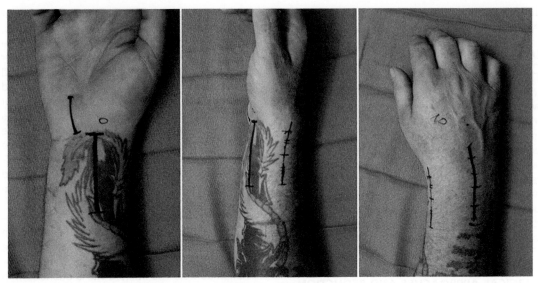

Fig. 6. Surgical incision planning in high-energy distal radius fractures.

encourage the fragment in place. The volar rim fragment can be provisionally fixed with a K-wire and the reduction is assessed on fluoroscopic imaging. The tear drop angle provides a radiographic assessment of the articular reduction of the volar rim (**Fig. 7**). Often the assistant at the end of the table will extend the wrist to visualize the surgery, and in doing so makes the reduction nearly impossible. The reduction of the volar ulnar corner requires the wrist to be in flexion and retractors carefully placed to adequately visualize the reduction. After confirmation of anatomic reduction, the volar ulnar corner is stabilized with an appropriate fragment-specific implant (see later section).

With the volar ulnar corner fragment anatomically reduced and secured, attention is turned to the dorsal wrist to address the dorsal ulnar corner and wall. A dorsal incision is made in line with the third metacarpal from the carpometacarpal joint to a few centimeters proximal to the Lister tubercle (see **Fig. 6**). The extensor pollicis longus is opened and an ulnarly based extensor retinacular flap is created by dividing the septation between the 3 to 4 and 4 to 5 extensor compartments. A radiocarpal arthrotomy is made along the dorsal radiocarpal ligament and radioscaphoid capsule to visualize the entire articular surface of the radius (**Fig. 8**). At this point, the dorsal ulnar corner and dorsal wall fragments can be visualized. The cortical bone is thin in this area and avoiding periosteal stripping may be the difference between contending with a dorsal wall "fragment" and dorsal comminution. A synovectomy and joint irrigation allows for visualization of the articular surface. There is a paradox of visualization and fracture reduction: if the fracture line is easily

visualized, then the dorsal fragments are not adequately reduced. In this instance, the dorsal fragments are extended, giving the surgeon superior visualization. In their proper position, the dorsal wall extends distally past the volar rim and visualization of the fracture line is difficult.

Any free intra-articular fragments can be well visualized through this dorsal capsulotomy. These free intra-articular fragments can be reduced with a probe or tamped up from underneath the subchondral bone as is commonly performed with tibial plateau fractures. Structural bone graft such as cancellous bone chips can help to raft the fragment and prevent re-displacement. Specific implants have been designed to provide direct fixation of these fragments. However, with adequate reduction and bone grafting, fixation of

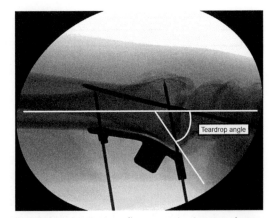

Fig. 7. Intraoperative fluoroscopic image demonstrating reduction of volar ulnar corner fragment with restoration of teardrop angle.

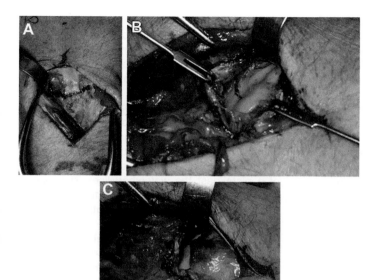

Fig. 8. A dorsal ligament sparing capsulotomy (*A*) allows direct visualization of the articular surface when the dorsal wall is not reduced (*B*). Anatomic dorsal wall reduction impedes visualization (*C*).

volar and dorsal fragments will often provide enough stability to the free intra-articular fragment.

Emphasizing again the importance of the lunate facet and sigmoid notch, the dorsal ulnar corner is the next fragment to be reduced. With the dorsal exposure already performed, direct reduction can be easily performed and a stable implant applied. The dorsal ulnar corner fragment is reduced and secured with an implant, followed by the intra-articular fragments and dorsal wall components(**Fig. 9**). Again, a final inspection of the articular surface will be difficult with the dorsal fragments adequately reduced. However, with retraction of the radial attachments of the dorsal radiocarpal ligament, wrist flexion, traction, and

the use of a headlight and freer elevator, the articular surface can be inspected to confirm adequate reduction.

Radial Column

The radial column can be visualized through an extended FCR approach or through a separate radial incision from the radial styloid extending just proximal to the outcroppers along the radial border. Alternatively, a longitudinal incision directly over the radial column can be made (see **Fig. 6**). Limiting subcutaneous dissection while maintaining skin perforators prevents skin necrosis between incisions, which is very uncommon.

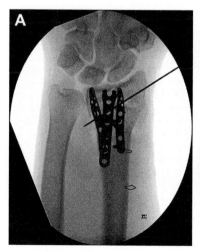
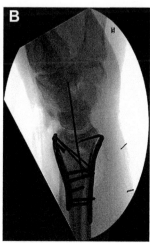

Fig. 9. AP (*A*) and lateral (*B*) intraoperative fluoroscopic images after application of dorsal fragment-specific implants to the dorsal ulnar corner and dorsal wall.

Care is taken to prevent injury to the radial sensory nerve branch. The fracture line often extends proximally to exit the radial cortex beneath the first extensor compartment. The distal 1 cm of the first extensor compartment retinaculum is maintained and the proximal portion is released to provide direct visualization of the fracture line and the extensor retinaculum of the compartment is preserved. The first extensor compartment tendons are retracted, identifying the transected brachioradialis tendon that was divided with the volar radius approach. The fracture is debrided of any remaining interposed soft tissue or fracture hematoma. Traction on the thumb, ulnar deviation, and direct manipulation of the fragment are usually sufficient to anatomically reduce the radial column. A K-wire started precisely on the bare area of the radial styloid just dorsal to the tendons and secured in the pedestal on the ulnar side of the radius provides provisional or definitive fixation. Anatomic reduction can be confirmed by returning to the dorsal incision and capsulotomy and directly visualizing the articular surface. Often the sagittal split remains visible until the radial column construct is applied and secured (**Fig. 10**).

IMPLANT CHOICES FOR THE RADIUS

The size of the fracture fragment determines the type of implant used for definitive fixation. A sagittal CT slice through the lunate facet is a good preoperative indication of the fragment size and ability to use a volar locking plate (**Fig. 11**). A volar locking plate is the first choice, as it affords the greatest stability to resist shear forces as a buttress. Standard volar plates have the advantage of a proven track record for certain fracture types and provide strong buttress support to volar

shear-type fractures. When metadiaphyseal comminution and bone loss is present, several of these volar locking plates have extended length options to bridge fracture gaps (**Fig. 12**). In some instances, dual plating with a volar locking plate and a standard 3.5-mm plate may be required to stabilize severe metadiaphyseal injuries. However, many high-energy distal radius fractures have small volar ulnar corner fragments that are too distal and too small to be secured by a volar locking plate safely (ie, requires very distal placement of a plate past the watershed line). The use of K-wires combined with volar plating has been described, but provide less rotational stability than fixed angled devices.[19]

In addition to volar locking plates, fragment-specific implants, bridge plates, and external fixation, with or without additional K-wire fixation have all been used for the treatment of these injuries. The advantage of fragment-specific implants in comminuted high-energy distal radius fractures is that they allow for stable fixation and are designed such that multiple implants can be placed to address other fragments without running out of room for stable fixation to the pedestal.

This highlights the benefit of low-profile fragment-specific implants to stabilize the volar ulnar corner or at most provisionally fixation of the volar ulnar corner before reduction of the free intra-articular and dorsal fragments. With a standard volar locking plate and a distal row of screws in place to secure a volar rim fragment, there is little ability to manipulate the remaining fragments of the intermediate column and achieve anatomic reduction. The proximity of dorsal ulnar corner and wall fragments to the extensor tendons requires that any implants placed distally must be low profile to avoid tendon irritation. Depending

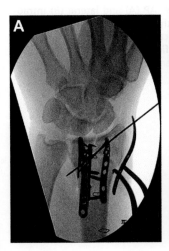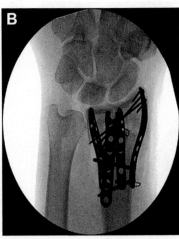

Fig. 10. AP intraoperative fluoroscopic images before (*A*) and after (*B*) fixation of the radial column plate.

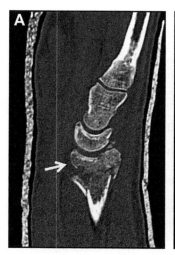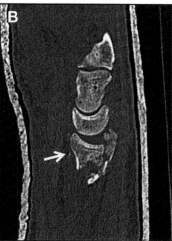

Fig. 11. Sagittal CT slices through the lunate fossa of high-energy distal radius fractures with small (*A*) and large (*B*) volar ulnar corner fragments. *Arrows* are pointing to the volar ulnar corner fragments.

on the implants used, a second implant may be placed specifically for the dorsal wall fragment.

A low-profile plate designed for the radial column can serve as a buttress to resist proximal displacement of the fragment. It is important to have a good familiarity with any implant placed on the radial column, as it is the most likely to cause extensor tendon or other soft tissue irritation and require hardware removal.[20] However, proximal and radial displacement of the styloid is common and a radial column plate is an excellent option to counter these deforming forces.

Bridge plates and external fixators disrupt the soft tissue minimally and are often used with indirect fracture reduction methods. It is important not to ignore the principles of periarticular fixation and bypass them with application of a bridge plate

because it might be easier. In our practice, the bridge plate is used as an adjunct to fragment-specific fixation, not in lieu of. For example, use of a bridge plate does not preclude a volar incision to reduce the volar rim and place a fragment-specific implant.

TREATMENT OF THE ULNAR COLUMN

Ulnar styloid fractures are no longer routinely fixed unless there is instability, which is not amenable to splinting.[21] Examination of the contralateral side should be used as a reference. Some high-energy distal radius fractures can be associated with challenging ulna fractures, including comminuted ulnar head fractures and distal ulnar shaft fractures. Dorsal-palmar stability of the ulna within

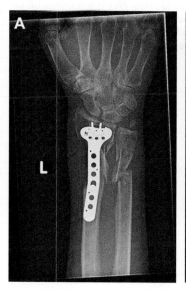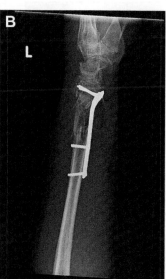

Fig. 12. PA (*A*) and lateral (*B*) intraoperative radiographs better visualize the bow of the radius in a high-energy distal radius fracture with metadiaphyseal comminution.

the sigmoid notch in full wrist protonation, supination, and neutral position is tested. Any excessive translation is suspect to loss of integrity of the foveal attachment of the TFCC. Alternatively, a forearm squeeze test can be performed. Under posterior to anterior fluoroscopy, the DRUJ is evaluated. Static image followed by an image with squeezing the interval between the radius and ulna in the forearm is undertaken. If the DRUJ space widens with the squeeze, a disruption of the fovea is suspected.

Surgical Approach and Reduction Techniques

An incision can be made over the subcutaneous border of the ulna from the ulnar styloid extending proximally below the fracture line. Care is taken to preserve ulnar sensory nerve branches. The interval between the extensor carpi ulnaris and flexor carpi ulnaris tendons yields direct access to the ulnar shaft to identify a fracture or repair an unstable TFCC.

If the TFCC is detached from the fovea, the preceding approach can be used for placing a suture anchor in the fovea, or alternatively the fifth compartment approach can be used from a dorsal approach, depending on the surgeon's comfort.

Implant Choices for the Ulna

For ulnar styloid fractures with instability, K-wire fixation with a tension band provides a low-profile construct. In more proximal fractures, the objective is to permit stable pronosupination and there is little need for 3.5-mm plates for fracture fixation, as is commonly used in midforearm ulnar

shaft fractures. Further, the short distal segment is often better managed with K-wires, fixed angled devices, or distal locking screws. Again, low-profile implants here have the benefit of less soft tissue irritation while maintaining length, alignment, and rotation.

FINAL ASSESSMENT

After all implants have been placed, intraoperative fluoroscopy of the wrist is performed, including anteroposterior (AP), lateral, and 15-degree tilt lateral to assess the articular surface. Reversing the fluoroscopy machine and obtaining a PA gives an alternative view of the articular with a slight change in orientation and projections to combat anchoring bias after viewing several AP images of the same fracture throughout the case. For comminuted metadiaphyseal fractures, an intraoperative plain film of the forearm is obtained to assess the overall bow of the radius. Last, live fluoroscopy can be used to assess the stability of the fracture construct with the wrist in flexion, extension, and radial and ulnar deviation. This final assessment of stability helps to formulate a plan for length of postoperative immobilization and commencement of early range of motion. If there is any concern about radiocarpal instability, fragment-specific fixation does not preclude the use of a bridge plate or external fixator for high-energy distal radius fractures.

Wounds are closed with interrupted nonabsorbable sutures. Careful surgical dissection, respecting perforators, and understanding the

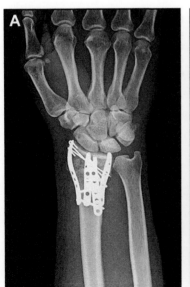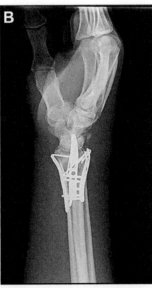

Fig. 13. Final PA (*A*) and lateral (*B*) radiographs of high-energy distal radius fracture treated with fragment-specific fixation.

angiosomes of the wrist have safely allowed multiple longitudinal incisions around the wrist. A mildly compressive wrap is placed around the sterile dressings for edema control, and the patient is placed in either a sugar tong splint or volar resting splint depending on the DRUJ assessment. Postoperatively, patients are encouraged to continue elevation, icing, and finger range of motion in addition to a multimodal pain regimen (**Fig. 13**).

SUMMARY

In some distal radius fractures, the mechanism of injury imparts enough injury to fracture subchondral bone and articular surfaces. Anatomic reduction requires attention to individual fragments that are too small or too distal to be stably fixed with standard volar locked plating. With the advent of low-profile fragment-specific implants, an algorithmic approach to open reduction internal fixation is possible. Emphasis is first placed on the volar rim and dorsal ulnar corner, as they make up 2 critical articular surfaces: the radiolunate and DRUJ. Anatomic reduction and stable fixation of individual fragments allows for early range of motion with low risk of hardware and wound complications.

CLINICS CARE POINTS

- Traction films can reveal small, intra-articular fracture fragments that may be difficult to identify after closed reduction and splinting is performed.

- A sagittal CT slice through the lunate facet is a good preoperative indication of the volar ulnar fragment size and ability to use a volar locking plate.

- The column model, which organizes the distal radius into an intermediate column, radial column, and pedestal, as well as a separate column for the ulna, provides a systematic approach to addressing these injuries

- Application of a fragment-specific approach uses multiple incisions that are strategically placed to address the major fragments of the distal radius fracture.

- Anatomic reduction and stable fixation of individual fragments allows for early range of motion with low risk of hardware and wound complications.

DISCLOSURE

A.Y. Shin: Royalties TriMed/Mayo Medical Ventures. N. Pulos: TriMed-honorarium.

REFERENCES

1. Nellans KW, Kowalski E, Chung KC. The epidemiology of distal radius fractures. Hand Clin 2012; 28(2):113–25.
2. Leversedge FJ, Srinivasan RC. Management of soft-tissue injuries in distal radius fractures. Hand Clin 2012;28(2):225–33.
3. Mandziak DG, Watts AC, Bain GI. Ligament contribution to patterns of articular fractures of the distal radius. J Hand Surg Am 2011;36(10): 1621–5.
4. Rhee SH, Baek GH. A correlation exists between subchondral bone mineral density of the distal radius and systemic bone mineral density. Clin Orthop Relat Res 2012;470(6):1682–9.
5. Pidgeon TS, DaSilva KA, Crisco JJ, et al. Three-dimensional characterization of trabecular bone mineral density of the distal radius utilizing quantitative computed tomography. Hand (N Y) 2020;15(1): 131–9.
6. Wæver D, Madsen ML, Rölfing JHD, et al. Distal radius fractures are difficult to classify. Injury 2018; 49(Suppl 1):S29–32.
7. Melone CP Jr. Articular fractures of the distal radius. Orthop Clin North Am 1984;15(2):217–36.
8. Frykman G. Fracture of the distal radius including sequelae–shoulder-hand-finger syndrome, disturbance in the distal radio-ulnar joint and impairment of nerve function. A clinical and experimental study. Acta Orthop Scand 1967;(Suppl 108):3+.
9. Jupiter JB, Fernandez DL. Comparative classification for fractures of the distal end of the radius. J Hand Surg Am 1997;22(4):563–71.
10. Medoff RJ. Essential radiographic evaluation for distal radius fractures. Hand Clin 2005;21(3): 279–88.
11. Lafontaine M, Hardy D, Delince P. Stability assessment of distal radius fractures. Injury 1989;20(4): 208–10.
12. Teunis T, Meijer S, Jupiter J, et al. The correlation between the teardrop angle and anterior lunate facet displacement in plating distal radial fractures. J Hand Surg Eur 2019;44(5):462–7.
13. Azi ML, Teixeira MB, de Carvalho SF, et al. Computed tomography vs standard radiograph in preoperative planning of distal radius fractures with articular involvement. Strategies Trauma Limb Reconstr 2019;14(1):15–9.
14. Levin LS, Rozell JC, Pulos N. Distal radius fractures in the elderly. J Am Acad Orthop Surg 2017;25(3): 179–87.

15. Howard M, Curtis A, Everett S, et al. Does a delay in surgery for distal radial fractures affect patient outcome? J Hand Surg Eur 2021;46(1):69–74.

16. Vincent S, Paskey T, Critchlow E, et al. Prospective randomized study examining preoperative opioid counseling on postoperative opioid consumption after upper extremity surgery. Hand (N Y) 2020. https://doi.org/10.1177/1558944720919936. 1558944720919936.

17. Rhee PC, Medoff RJ, Shin AY. Complex distal radius fractures: an anatomic algorithm for surgical management. J Am Acad Orthop Surg 2017;25(2):77–88.

18. Hara T, Horii E, An KN, et al. Force distribution across wrist joint: application of pressure-sensitive conductive rubber. J Hand Surg Am 1992;17(2):339–47.

19. Moore AM, Dennison DG. Distal radius fractures and the volar lunate facet fragment: Kirschner wire fixation in addition to volar-locked plating. Hand (N Y) 2014;9(2):230–6.

20. Galle SE, Harness NG, Hacquebord JH, et al. Complications of radial column plating of the distal radius. Hand (N Y) 2019;14(5):614–9.

21. Mulders MAM, Fuhri Snethlage LJ, de Muinck Keizer RO, et al. Functional outcomes of distal radius fractures with and without ulnar styloid fractures: a meta-analysis. J Hand Surg Eur 2018;43(2):150–7.

Arthroscopy in Distal Radius Fractures
Indications and When to Do It

Jeffrey Yao, MD*, Nathaniel Fogel, MD

KEYWORDS

- Distal radius • Fracture • Wrist arthroscopy • Interosseus ligament injuries • TFCC

KEY POINTS

- Wrist arthroscopy in the setting of distal radius fracture allows for direct visualization of reduction of the articular surface and identification and treatment of associated soft tissue injuries.
- Arthroscopy should be considered in intra-articular fractures with residual step-off or gap of greater than 2 mm after traditional reduction techniques particularly in the young, active patient.
- Arthroscopic techniques are particularly useful for addressing free articular fragments and die-punch lesions, and to address rotational malreductions.
- Level I evidence supporting the use of arthroscopy in treatment of intra-articular distal radius fractures is limited, and studies investigating functional outcomes report mixed results with its use.

INTRODUCTION

Having first gained popularity as a treatment adjunct for distal radius fractures (DRFs) in the 1990s, wrist arthroscopy represents a unique tool to treat injuries to the distal radial articular surface and associated soft tissues of the wrist.[1–8] One of the fundamental principles of treatment for intra-articular fractures is anatomic reduction of the joint surface, of which arthroscopy provides an unparalleled view. The importance of anatomic reduction in DRF is well established. Knirk and Jupiter[9] reported radiographic evidence of post-traumatic arthritis in 91% of patients with residual joint incongruity after DRF as opposed to just 11% in those who healed without radiographic joint incongruity, and found arthrosis was present in 100% of patients with a residual step-off or gap of greater than 2 mm. The degree of postoperative step-off and gap has also been shown to be correlated with functional outcome,[10] although this remains controversial.[11]

Direct arthroscopic visualization has been established to be more accurate than fluoroscopy in assessing articular step-off or gap.[12–15] In a representative study, Abe and colleagues[16] reported on 118 wrists with intra-articular DRFs of which 108 appeared to achieve reduction on fluoroscopy alone, only to find that 38 of those wrists had persistent step-off or gap of greater than 2 mm on examination under arthroscopy. Omokawa and colleagues[17] reported similar results, noting that 88 of 273 wrists (22%) had persistent step-off or gap of more than 2 mm after reduction under fluoroscopy was thought to be sufficient. Malreduction in the sagittal plane can be particularly difficult to assess on plain radiographs alone, given overlapping densities from ulna, scaphoid, and lunate fossa artifact present on the lateral view.[18]

Arthroscopy also affords the opportunity to identify and subsequently address associated soft tissue injuries, particularly to the scapholunate interosseous ligament (SLIL), lunotriquetral

Department of Orthopaedic Surgery, Stanford University Medical Center, 540 Broadway Street MC 6342, Redwood City, CA 94063, USA
* Corresponding author.
E-mail address: jyao@stanford.edu

Hand Clin 37 (2021) 279–291
https://doi.org/10.1016/j.hcl.2021.02.010
0749-0712/21/© 2021 Elsevier Inc. All rights reserved.

interosseous ligament (LTIL), and triangular fibrocartilage complex (TFCC), which are common in intra-articular DRFs.[2,3,19] It also allows for removal of intra-articular hematoma and joint debris without compromising the integrity of the capsule or stability of the radiocarpal joint.[20] This has historically been a proposed benefit for arthroscopic intervention; however, a recent level I randomized controlled trial (RCT) by Selles and colleagues[21] found no benefit as measured by Disability of Arm Shoulder and Hand (DASH) questionnaire, patient-rated wrist evaluation, pain scores, wrist range of motion (ROM), or grip strength in those who underwent arthroscopy for the purpose of hematoma evacuation at time of internal fixation for DRF.

Despite its proposed benefits, arthroscopic-assisted techniques are not widely used. Wrist arthroscopy has a learning curve and may be thought to be cumbersome, time-consuming, and/or challenging by lower-volume arthroscopists. Surgical times are increased in comparison with fluoroscopic-assisted procedures, and arthroscopy is associated with increased cost and use of resources. The American Academy of Orthopaedic Surgeons Clinical Practice Guidelines for Treatment of DRFs supports only weak recommendations for arthroscopic evaluation of the joint surface at the time of surgical fixation; surgical treatment of SLIL, LTIL, and TFCC tears at the time of surgical fixation; and for the use of wrist arthroscopy to improve accuracy of diagnosis of intercarpal ligament injuries based on the available literature.[22] Although the merit of arthroscopy in its ability to assess the articular surface and evaluate soft tissue injuries is accepted, understanding exactly when and how to use this tool remains unclear to many practicing hand surgeons. We aim to provide an evidence-based framework to better elucidate how to best incorporate wrist arthroscopy in the setting of DRF.

INDICATIONS AND CONTRAINDICATIONS
Fracture Characteristics

To date, proponents of arthroscopy in the setting of treatment of DRFs have cited intra-articular step-off or gap of greater than 2 mm seen on radiographs as the primary indication for the utilization of the technique (**Fig. 4**).[23,24] Some studies suggest the threshold for articular step-off or gap should be 1 mm.[25] Patient age, medical comorbidities, and level of activity should be considered before proceeding with surgical intervention. Arthroscopy may be used before initial reduction techniques or may be used after provisional reduction under fluoroscopy has been performed. Our

preference is to perform soft tissue releases (ie, the brachioradialis) and perform provisional reduction maneuvers before using arthroscopy to "fine tune" our intra-articular reduction. Once the reduction is optimized, stabilization and fixation is performed by using volar locked plates, fragment-specific implants, external fixation, percutaneous Kirschner-wire (K-wire) fixation, and/or dorsal spanning plates, depending on, for example, the severity of the fracture or size and stability of the fragments.

Fractures of the radial styloid (**Fig. 1**), displaced 3-part and 4-part fractures, as well as fractures involving central articular or "die-punch" fragment are patterns particularly amenable to arthroscopic techniques and are our most common indications for using arthroscopy.[26] Malrotation of the radial styloid may be easily missed on fluoroscopic evaluation.[27] Provisional reduction may be obtained under fluoroscopy after the deforming soft tissues are released and then confirmed and "fine-tuned" via arthroscopy (**Fig. 2**). Fractures of the radial styloid are best evaluated with the arthroscope in the 6-R portal.[27] Definitive fixation may be obtained with K-wires or cannulated headless compression screws (**Fig. 3**). Displaced 3-part and 4-part fractures may be addressed after reducing the radial styloid fragment as described previously, and using the radial styloid fragment as a template off of which to gauge the reduction of the other fragments.

Concomitant Injuries

Intra-articular DRFs are highly associated with intercarpal ligamentous pathology, particularly injury to the SLIL and LTIL, as well as TFCC injuries. Arthroscopic-assisted fixation for DRF provides the added benefit of being able to diagnose these injuries, as well as have the opportunity to treat them acutely. Arthroscopy is the standard for evaluation of these injuries, as preoperative radiographs have been shown to have poor predictive indicators of interosseus ligament injury, particularly of the SLIL, and acute MRI in the setting of fracture is rarely used.[6,24] Richards and colleagues[6] reported on 118 acute intra-articular and extra-articular DRFs and found that at time of arthroscopic evaluation, 60% of all SLIL injuries had normal preoperative radiographs, whereas 50% of those with a widened scapholunate interval of more than 3 mm had no ligamentous injury. Culp and Osterman[3] reported on 27 patients with intra-articular DRFs who underwent arthroscopic-assisted reduction and fixation, and found 55% of patients had concomitant SLIL injury, 23% had LTIL injury, 42% had a TFCC

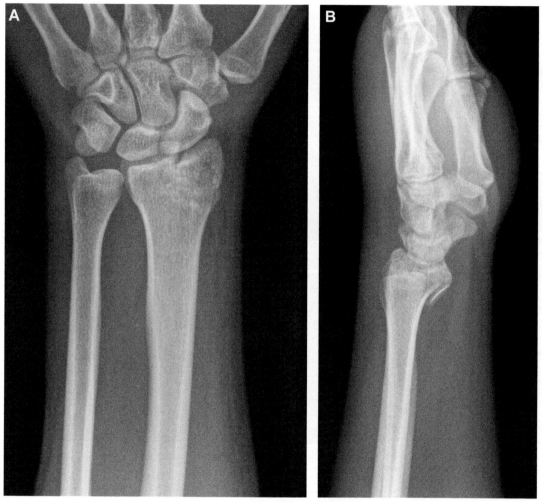

Fig. 1. Posterior-anterior (*A*) and lateral (*B*) radiographs of an intra-articular DRF with greater than 2 mm of intra-articular step-off.

tear, and 42% had carpal chondral injuries. Lindau and colleagues[7] performed wrist arthroscopy in 50 displaced DRFs and all but 1 case found an associated ligamentous injury, with the TFCC being involved in 78% of cases. A review of associated injuries across 13 studies from 1995 to 2009 reported similar data, with SLIL injuries present in 45%, TFCC injuries in 50%, and chondral injuries in 29% of DRFs.[19]

Although the presence of associated injuries and the ability to identify them on arthroscopy is well documented, the indications to intervene acutely on this pathology are not as widely agreed on. Swart and Tang[19] evaluated 42 patients with DRF and cataloged soft tissue injuries at time of initial fixation. They reported no significant difference in DASH scores, visual analogue scale pain rating, ROM, and radiographic outcomes between subjects with and without associated soft tissue

injuries at 1 year. All patients underwent internal fixation with volar locked plating and progressed through the same postoperative protocol. Mrkonjic and colleagues[28] reported similar results with 13-year follow-up on 51 patients who sustained DRF, of whom 32 had concomitant grade I to III SLIL injuries that were not treated at time of original arthroscopic assessment. They found no difference in any significant subjective, objective, or radiographic measures collected. It is important to note that this study did not include any grade IV injuries.[28] A review of the same cohort also reported no significant difference in outcomes for patients with partial or complete TFCC injuries that was not addressed as compared with those who did not have any TFCC injury.[29] Only 1 patient with a TFCC injury ultimately underwent a second procedure to address subsequently symptomatic distal radioulnar joint (DRUJ) instability. Although

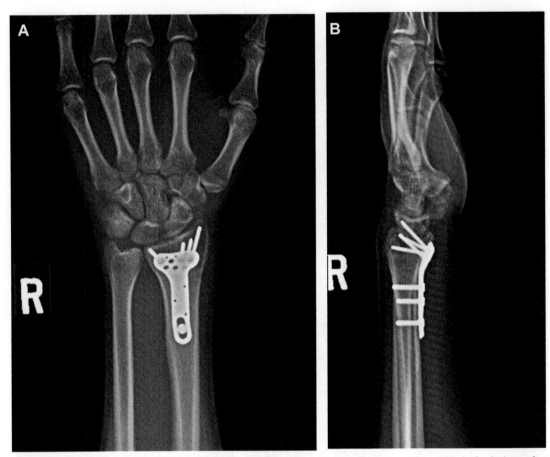

Fig. 2. Posterior-anterior (*A*) and lateral (*B*) radiographs demonstrating fixation with a volar locked plate after reduction under arthroscopic assistance.

level 1 or 2 evidence supporting acute intervention for most soft tissue injuries in the setting of DRFs is lacking, many investigators advocate treating severe intercarpal ligament and complete TFCC tears at the time of fracture fixation based on smaller series and clinical experience.[4,5,26,30]

Wrist arthroscopy has also been described to aid in assessing when ulnar styloid fractures are indicated for fixation. Although the presence of an ulnar styloid fracture in and of itself is not an indication for arthroscopy-assisted techniques, direct evaluation allows for evaluation of laxity of the TFCC and DRUJ after fixation of the DRF.[27] In the setting of residual DRUJ laxity after the presence of a peripheral TFCC tear has been ruled out, stabilization of the ulnar styloid may be indicated.

Contraindications

Contraindications to an arthroscopic-assisted approach include a significant capsular injury, infection, abnormal anatomy that would preclude safe portal placement, and neurovascular injury.[26] Extravasation concerns, as well as prior issues associated with open fractures, may be avoided by performing dry arthroscopy as described by del Piñal and colleagues.[31] It is important to note that some described contraindications to isolated arthroscopic reduction and percutaneous fixation, such as carpal tunnel symptoms or preexisting compartment syndrome, do not preclude arthroscopy being used as an adjunct to volar plating or other open treatment modalities.[32]

PREOPERATIVE PLANNING
Radiographic Workup

Preoperative radiographs should be obtained and scrutinized for suspicion of significant intra-articular step-off or gap, as well as evidence of associated intercarpal injuries. Some investigators recommend routinely obtaining preoperative computed tomography (CT) scans with or without 3-dimensional reconstruction for surgical planning.[24] CT has been shown to be superior to plain radiographs in elucidating involvement of the DRUJ, die-punch fragments, and the extent of comminution.[33] It is important to emphasize that

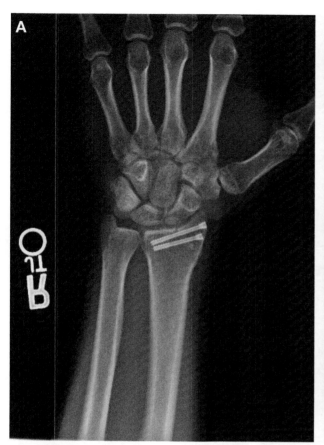
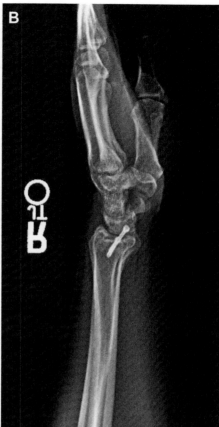

Fig. 3. Posterior-anterior (*A*) and lateral (*B*) radiographs demonstrating fixation of a displaced radial styloid fracture using cannulated headless compression screws after reduction under arthroscopic assistance.

central articular fragments have no ligamentous attachment and will not benefit from ligamentotaxis associated with closed reduction.[26] The presence and/or orientation of these central fragments are difficult to assess on plain radiographs. In our opinion, these types of fractures are the best indication for the use of adjunctive arthroscopy. CT has its limitations as well, as in one study free fracture fragments not appreciated on preoperative imaging were found at the time of arthroscopy in 9% of displaced intra-articular fractures.[17] In highly comminuted fractures, CT may be useful in identifying the largest articular fragment to which one can build back the articular surface. This segment may be fixed to a volar locking plate and then used as a reference for arthroscopic reduction of the remaining fragments.[34]

Ono and colleagues[35] reported a novel technique for using preoperative imaging to better understand which intra-articular DRFs may benefit from arthroscopically assisted reduction versus those that would result in residual articular step-off or gap of less than 2 mm. They suggest using a cutoff value of the sum of the

preoperative articular displacement on a plain lateral radiograph and coronal CT of 5.8 mm. In their series, this metric would have indicated the need for arthroscopic evaluation of all fractures that ended up with unacceptable step-off or gap after fixation with volar locked plating under fluoroscopy, whereas only overindicating approximately 17% of fractures that would have ultimately achieved sufficient reduction under fluoroscopy alone.[35]

That all being said, we have not felt that the routine use of CT scans for every DRF is necessary, and typically use it only for the most highly comminuted, complex intra-articular fractures.

Timing

There is relative consensus that the ideal time for arthroscopic-assisted DRF fixation should be within 3 to 7 days of injury.[2,3,23] Intervening acutely within the first 72 hours of the injury may be complicated by bleeding as well as increased fluid extravasation into the soft tissues if using wet arthroscopy. Mobilization of fracture fragments

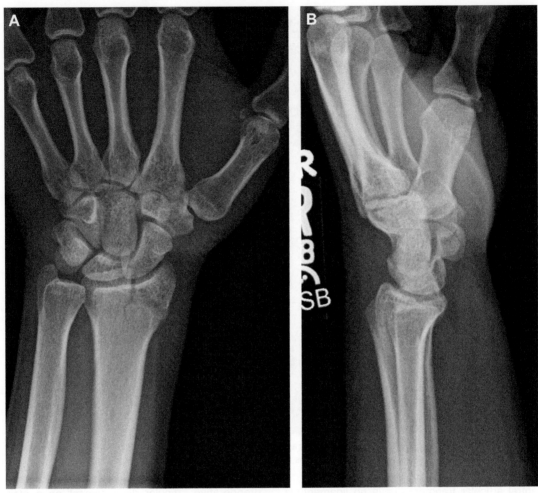

Fig. 4. Posterior-anterior (*A*) and lateral (*B*) radiographs of an intra-articular DRF with greater than 2 mm of intra-articular gapping.

using arthroscopic techniques becomes difficult beyond 1 week after the injury. It is important to note, however, that delayed presentation does not preclude the use of this technique, as it has been described in the treatment of distal radius malunion.[36]

PROCEDURAL APPROACH
Patient Positioning

The patient is positioned supine with the arm supported on a hand table. A pneumatic tourniquet is placed on the operative arm with care taken to be proximal enough avoid interfering with the arthroscopy tower setup. An Esmarch elastic bandage is used to exsanguinate the limb before tourniquet inflation. The extremity is then placed into the wrist arthroscopy tower with 12 to 15 pounds of longitudinal traction placed on the index and long fingers.

Surgical Technique

- Wrist arthroscopy may be performed at the outset of the procedure, after initial open exposure in the setting of planned dorsal or volar plating, or after a provisional reduction and fixation. This is completely based on the fracture pattern and mobility of the fragments. We prefer performing the wrist arthroscopy first unless there are soft tissue releases (ie, brachioradialis; dorsal periosteum) that must be performed beforehand to release the deforming forces on the fragments. In isolated die-punch fragments unattached to any deforming soft tissues (ie, the lunate facet), arthroscopic reduction may be performed before any soft tissue releases.
- Establish the 3 to 4, 6R, and mid-carpal portals and perform a standard diagnostic arthroscopy (**Fig. 5**). Arthroscopy may be

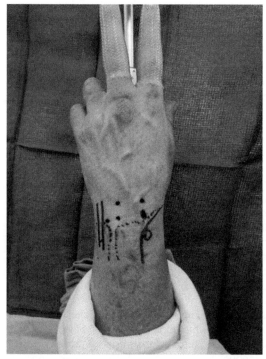

Fig. 5. Arthroscopic setup with relevant anatomy marked (long extensor tendon tendon, Lister tubercle, distal radius, distal ulna, DRUJ, extensor carpi ulnaris) to aid in accurately establishing portals.

performed dry or with very minimal fluid ("moist arthroscopy") via gravity-fed delivery to minimize extravasation into the soft tissues. The fractures are identified and any associated intercarpal ligament or TFCC injuries are identified and treated if necessary.

- A 3.5-mm shaver is used to debride and remove the associated hematoma and radiocarpal hemarthrosis (**Figs. 6** and **7**).The freer

elevator, probe, dental pick, trochar, osteotome, or the shaver itself may be used to manipulate each fragment. K-wire fixation is useful both as a way to manipulate fragments as well as hold provisional fixation after arthroscopic reduction.

- Abe and colleagues[16] describe a plate presetting arthroscopic reduction technique, in which fracture fragments are provisionally reduced using manipulation and pinning under fluoroscopy. A small volar incision is made by using the interval between flexor carpi radialis and the radial artery. All soft tissue releases as needed are performed. A volar locking plate is then preset to the volar diaphysis of the radius before suspending the wrist in traction for the wrist arthroscopy. Arthroscopy is performed through standard dorsal portals, and the existing volar wound is used to safely access the volar portal, allowing for visualization and evaluation of dorsal pathology. Residual step-off or gapping is then corrected under direct visualization before fixation with the volar plate is completed. Del Piñal and colleagues[31] describe a similar technique in which a provisional reduction is obtained through standard measures with manual manipulation and fixation of a volar locking plate and optimized under fluoroscopy before fine tuning the reduction under direct visualization (**Fig. 8**).
- Radial styloid fractures may be addressed via the use of a K-wire as a joystick in the unstable segment. The reduction is best assessed with the arthroscope in the 6R portal. The K-wire used for reduction may also serve as the guidewire for cannulated screw fixation (**Fig. 9**A–F).

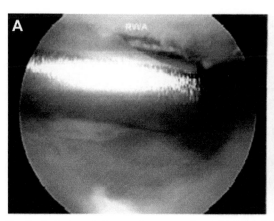
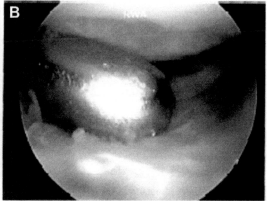

Fig. 6. Arthroscopic image demonstrating initial debridement (A) and reduction (B) of an intra-articular gap between the scaphoid and lunate facets of the distal radius articular surface.

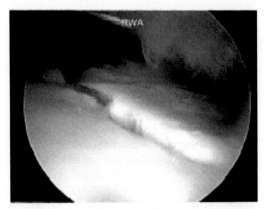

Fig. 7. Arthroscopic view demonstrating intra-articular step-off after completion of debridement.

- Arthroscopy is particularly useful in addressing articular fragments with rotated "upside-down articular fragments."[24] The orientation of the fragment is often missed on fluoroscopy alone, and even if identified on preoperative imaging are challenging to reorient without manipulation under direct visualization (**Fig. 10**).
- For mobile central articular fragments, there is often a subchondral void that will result in settling below the surrounding articular surface after reduction is achieved. In this case, screws or smooth pegs may be placed into the accompanying volar locked plate and the overlying fragment is impacted down on top of the implants with or without the addition of bone graft or bone graft substitute. The underlying implants will prevent depression of the joint surface.[26]

OUTCOMES

There is an absence of level I studies directly addressing the benefit of or lack thereof with regard to functional outcomes associated with arthroscopic-assisted reduction and fixation.[24] Among a collection of smaller prospective and retrospective studies, outcomes data are mixed. A systematic review by Smeraglia and colleagues[37] identified multiple issues with the existing outcomes literature, namely a scarcity of high-quality RCTs involving the use of volar locked plating and poor stratification of patient demographic data within existing studies, particularly patient age and fracture characteristics.

In a systematic review of the literature from 2006 to 2017 by Saab and colleagues,[38] 3 of the more relevant questions related to the use of arthroscopy in treating DRFs were investigated: does it improve articular reduction, how does it impact diagnosis and treatment of associated injuries, and how does it impact functional outcomes. Thirteen of the 16 studies reviewed noted the benefit of arthroscopy in attaining a more anatomic reduction of the joint surface, and importantly included studies that implemented volar locked plating as well as other methods of fixation. Of the 12 studies investigating the diagnosis and treatment of interosseous ligament and TFCC injuries, only 2 studies were comparative in nature. Eight of the 12 studies ultimately reported a positive contribution of arthroscopy, concluding that early diagnosis and intervention improved patient outcomes. Finally, conclusions from studies assessing functional outcomes were mixed. Of the 12 studies reviewed, only 6 reported positive outcomes with the use of arthroscopy. Of note, only 3 of the 12 were conducted prospectively.

Further evaluation of comparative studies supports the preceding findings. Yamazaki and colleagues[39] reported on 74 patients with unstable intra-articular DRFs randomized to fluoroscopic versus arthroscopic-assisted fixation with volar locked plating and found no significant difference

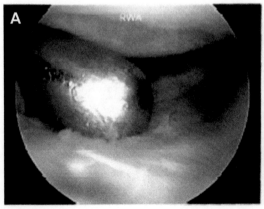
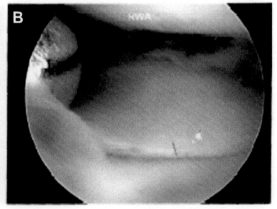

Fig. 8. Arthroscopic image demonstrating reduction with a blunt trochar (*A*) and subsequent anatomic reduction (*B*).

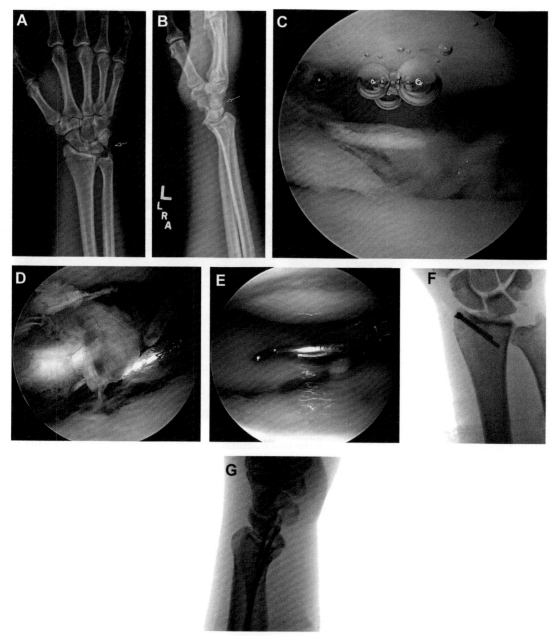

Fig. 9. (*A, B*) Posterior-anterior (PA) (*A*) and lateral (*B*) injury radiographs demonstrating a displaced intra-articular involving the radial styloid. (*C*) Arthroscopic image demonstrating step-off at the articular surface. A probe is used to mobilize and debride (*D*), and subsequently used to obtain and temporarily hold the anatomic reduction (*E*). PA (*F*) and lateral (*G*) fluoroscopic images demonstrating cannulated screw fixation. The screws were placed over the original wires used to aid in the initial arthroscopic-assisted reduction.

in radiographic step-off or gap, radial inclination, volar angulation, ulnar variance, or DASH scores. Although prior literature reported good outcomes with arthroscopy in the setting of fixation with pins or an external fixator, Yamazaki and colleagues[39] hypothesized that volar locked plating and the benefits it affords, including early mobilization and fixed angle fixation, limits the additional benefit offered from direct visualization via the arthroscope. Saab and colleagues[38] reported on preoperative and postoperative articular step and gap as measured by CT scan, and found no significant difference between those who underwent arthroscopic-assisted osteosynthesis

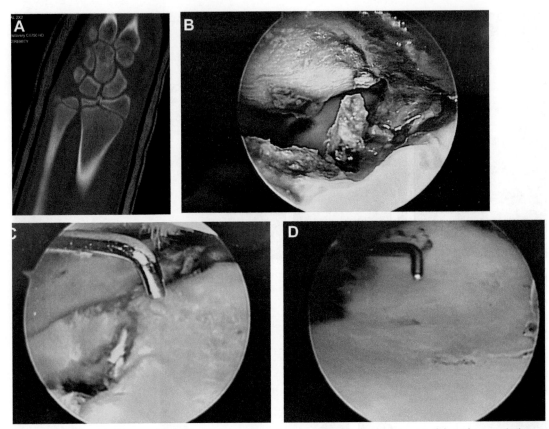

Fig. 10. (*A*) Coronal CT scan demonstrating a malrotated central articular fragment. (*B*) Arthroscopic image demonstrating articular gapping demonstrating the free malrotated central fragment. (*C*) A probe is used to obtain incremental reduction after excision of the central fragment. (*D*) Final reduction of the articular surface.

and those who did not. They also found no difference in clinical outcomes at 1-year follow-up.

In contrast, Varitimidis and colleagues[13] performed a prospective study of arthroscopic plus fluoroscopic-assisted fixation versus fluoroscopic-assisted alone in 40 patients with C-type DRFs with more than 2 mm of articular step-off or gap after closed reduction. They reported decreased pain and an earlier return to daily activities in the arthroscopy-assisted group, as well as statistically significant improvements in ROM in supination, extension, and flexion at 1-year follow-up. Mehta and colleagues[18] reported a series of 31 intra-articular DRFs treated with arthroscopically assisted reduction. They found that postoperative radiographic step-off was significantly correlated with pain, with patients with no step-off or less than 1-mm step-off reporting an incidence of 18% and 38%, respectively, as compared with 100% incidence in those with 2-mm step-off. They were able to obtain less than 1 mm in radiographic step-off in 86% of patients using arthroscopic-assisted technique, with 88% of patients reporting good to excellent New York

Orthopedic Hospital scores. Ruch and colleagues[40] reported on outcomes of 15 patients who underwent fluoroscopically assisted reduction and external fixation versus 15 patients who underwent arthroscopically assisted reduction and external fixation for intra-articular DRF. Those in the arthroscopic-assisted group reported statistically significantly superior supination, wrist extension, and wrist flexion compared with the fluoroscopy group, but no difference in radiographic metrics or DASH scores at final follow-up.

Abe and Fujii[41] report a series of 248 intra-articular DRFs treated with arthroscopic-assisted techniques. Of 231 fractures thought to be sufficiently reduced under fluoroscopy, 49 were found to have residual step-off or gap of greater than 2 mm when examined arthroscopically, demonstrating the superiority of arthroscopy in assessing and obtaining anatomic reduction over fluoroscopy. At final follow-up, 98% reported a Mayo Modified Wrist Score of excellent or good, mean DASH was 3.4, and mean grip strength of 91.5% of the contralateral side. Although this study does not have a control group, it is notable within the literature for the number of subjects included and demonstrates consistently strong outcomes with this arthroscopically assisted technique.

COMPLICATIONS

Overall complication rates associated with wrist arthroscopy have been reported in the range of 4.7% to 6.0% in large review studies.[42,43] The most common complications include the failure to achieve the desired outcome, iatrogenic nerve and cartilage injuries, and complex regional pain syndrome. Stiffness, tendon injury, and postoperative hematoma are rare but reported complications.[32,42] There is a theoretic risk of compartment syndrome in the setting of DRF when fluid is used, particularly if driven by an automated pump.

One of the primary criticisms of wrist arthroscopy in the setting of DRF is the additional operative time needed and the associated learning curve with arthroscopy techniques. The literature supports the notion that low-volume wrist arthroscopists have a significantly higher complication rate associated with the procedure. Leclercq and colleagues[42] reported a significant inflection point in complication rate at the hands of surgeons performing fewer than 25 wrist arthroscopies annually as well as in those with less than 5 years of clinical practice experience (12.1% and 13.6% complication rates, respectively). This is compared with complication rates 5% and lower with higher volume and more experienced practitioners.

It is also important to note the increased operative time, cost, and utilization of resources associated with wrist arthroscopy.[13,44] Arthroscopic-assisted reduction techniques are not as easily applied by inexperienced surgeons.[24] When considering any given surgical technique, it is necessary to consider the familiarity of the given surgeon with that procedure and weigh the proposed benefit of the procedure against potential complications and resource utilization consequences.

CLINICS CARE POINTS

- The risk of associated soft tissue swelling or compartment syndrome may be avoided by proceeding with dry arthroscopy techniques if there is a particular concern in a given case. Capsular defects or open wounds are not absolute contraindications to using arthroscopic techniques.[31]
- Patients with residual intra-articular step-off or gap on fluoroscopy after standard

reduction techniques and open approaches may benefit from arthroscopic assistance in obtaining a more accurate reduction. Even if arthroscopy is not in the original operative plan, having it available if needed when starting a case with displaced articular components is beneficial.

- Arthroscopy is useful to validate radiographic findings both preoperatively and intraoperatively. Abe and Fujii[41] reported 9.3% of wrists in their series were found to have free fracture fragments that were not identified with preoperative plain radiographs or CT scans. In highly comminuted patterns, we have a lower threshold to move to direct visualization in lieu of relying on CT to look for the presence of these fragments. Intraoperatively, arthroscopy allows for confirmation that distal screws or pegs are not penetrating the joint space.
- Surgeon experience with wrist arthroscopy is essential for these techniques, as complication rates are significantly higher in lower-volume practitioners.[42]
- Outside of the most experienced arthroscopists, arthroscopic techniques should be reserved for fractures less than a week old, as mobilization of fragments and subsequent reduction becomes quite challenging outside of the acute setting.

SUMMARY

Use of arthroscopy in the setting of DRF fixation may play an instrumental role in assisting with reduction of residual step-off and gapping of intra-articular fractures, as well as identifying and treating associated soft tissue injuries. There is utility to this technique particularly in the setting of residual intra-articular displacement after reduction under fluoroscopy, in patterns with depressed central articular components, and in the presence of high-grade soft tissue injuries. Familiarity and comfort with wrist arthroscopy techniques may remain a barrier to wide adoption, but wrist arthroscopic techniques remain on the rise in hand fellowship training programs worldwide. Further investigation is needed to elucidate whether the improved accuracy in articular reduction attained with arthroscopy produces clinically meaningful functional outcomes over fractures treated without adjunctive arthroscopy.

DISCLOSURES

The authors have nothing to disclose.

REFERENCES

1. Whipple TL. The role of arthroscopy in the treatment of wrist injuries in the athlete. Clin Sports Med 1998; 17(3):623–34.

2. Geissler WB, Freeland AE, Savoie FH, et al. Intra-carpal soft tissue lesions associated with an intra-articular fracture of the distal end of the radius. J Bone Joint Surg Am 1996;78A:357–65.

3. Culp RW, Osterman AL. Arthroscopic reduction and internal fixation of distal radius fractures. Orthop Clin North Am 1995;26(4):739–48.

4. Ruch DS, Yang CC, Paterson Smith B. Results of acute arthroscopically repaired triangular fibrocarti-lage complex injuries associated with intra-articular distal radius fractures. Arthroscopy 2003;19:511–6.

5. Lindau T. Arthroscopic evaluation of associated soft tissue injuries in distal radius fractures. Hand Clin 2017;33(4):651–8.

6. Richards RS, Bennett JD, Roth JH, et al. Arthro-scopic diagnosis of intra-articular soft tissue injuries associated with distal radial fractures. J Hand Surg Am 1997;22:772–6.

7. Lindau T, Arner M, Hagberg L. Intraarticular lesions in distal fractures of the radius in young adults. A descriptive arthroscopic study in 50 patients. J Hand Surg Br 1997;22(5):638–43.

8. Fowler Timothy. Intercarpal ligament injuries associ-ated with distal radius fractures. J Am Acad Orthop Surg 2019;27(20):e893–901.

9. Knirk JL, Jupiter JB. Intra-articular fractures of the distal end of the radius in young adults. J Bone Joint Surg Am 1986;68(5):647–59.

10. Trumble TE, Schmitt SR, Vedder NB. Factors affecting functional outcome of displaced intra-articular distal radius fractures. J Hand Surg Am 1994;19:325–40.

11. Goldfarb CA, Rudzki JR, Catalano LW, et al. Fifteen-year outcome of displaced intra-articular fractures of the distal radius. J Hand Surg Am 2006;31(4):633–9.

12. Lutsky K, Boyer MI, Steffen JA, et al. Arthroscopic assessment of intra-articular distal radius fractures after open reduction and internal fixation from a volar approach. J Hand Surg Am 2008;33(4):476–84.

13. Varitimidis SE, Basdekis GK, Dialiana ZH, et al. Treatment of intra-articular fractures of the distal radius: Fluoroscopic or arthroscopic reduction? J Bone Joint Surg Br 2008;90(6):778–85.

14. Auge WK, Velazquez PA. The application of indirect reduction techniques in the distal radius: the role of adjuvant arthroscopy. Arthroscopy 2000;16:830–5.

15. Edwards CC, Haraszti CJ, McGillivary GR, et al. In-traarticular distal radius fractures: arthroscopic assessment of radiographically assisted reduction. J Hand Surg Am 2001;26(6):1036–41.

16. Abe Y, Yoshida K, Tominaga Y. Less invasive surgery with wrist arthroscopy for distal radius fracture. J Orthop Sci 2013;18(3):398–404.

17. Omokawa S, Abe Y, Imatani J, et al. Treatment of intra-articular distal radius fractures. Hand Clin 2017;33(3):529–43.

18. Mehta JA, Bain GI, Heptinstall RJ. Anatomical reduction of intra-articular fractures of the distal radius. An arthroscopically-assisted approach. J Bone Joint Surg Br 2000;82:79–86.

19. Swart E, Tang P. The effect of ligament injuries on out- comes of operatively treated distal radius frac-tures. Am J Orthop 2017;46(1):E41–6.

20. Doi K, Hattori Y, Otsuka K, et al. Intra-articular frac-tures of the distal aspect of the radius: arthroscopi-cally assisted reduction compared with open reduction and internal fixation. J Bone Joint Surg Am 1999;81:1093–110.

21. Selles CA, Mulders MAM, Colaris JW, et al. Arthro-scopic debridement does not enhance surgical treatment of intra-articular distal radius fractures: a randomized control trial. J Hand Surg Eur 2020; 45(4):327–32.

22. Lichtman DM, Bindra RR, Boyer MI, et al. Treatment of distal radius fractures. J Am Acad Orthop Surg 2010;18(3):180–9.

23. Abboudi J, Culp RW. Treating fractures of the distal radius with arthroscopic assistance. Orthop Clin North Am 2001;32(2):307–15.

24. Ardouin L, Durand A, Gay A, et al. Why do we use arthroscopy for distal radius fractures? Eur J Orthop Surg Traumatol 2018;28:1505–14.

25. Fernandez DL, Geissler WB. Treatment of displaced articular fractures of the radius. J Hand Surg Am 1991;16(3):375–84.

26. Slutsky DJ. Portals and methodology. In: del Pinal F, Mathoulin C, Luchetti R, editors. Arthroscopic man-agement of distal radius fractures. Berlin (Germany): Springer; 2007. p. 13–26.

27. Geissler WB. Intra-articular distal radius fractures: the role of arthroscopy? Hand Clin 2005;21(3):407–16.

28. Mrkonjic A, Lindau T, Geijer M, et al. Arthroscopi-cally diagnosed scapholunate ligament injuries associated with distal radial fractures: a 13- to 15-year follow-up. J Hand Surg Am 2015;40(6): 1077–82.

29. Mrkonjic A, Geijer M, Lindau T, et al. The natural course of traumatic triangular fibrocartilage complex tears in distal radial fractures: a 13-15 year follow-up of arthroscopically diagnosed but untreated injuries. J Hand Surg Am 2012;37(8):1555–60.

30. Kasapinova K, Kamiloski V. Influence of associated lesions of the intrinsic ligaments on distal radius fractures outcome. Arch Orthop Trauma Surg 2015;135(6):831–8.

31. del Piñal F, Garcia-Bernal FJ, Pisani D, et al. Dry arthroscopy of the wrist: surgical technique. J Hand Surg Am 2007;32:119–23.

32. Wiesler ER, Chloros GD, Lucas RM, et al. Arthro-scopic management of volar lunate facet fractures

of the distal radius. Tech Hand Up Extrem Surg 2006;10(3):139–44.

33. Pruitt DL, Gilula LA, Manske PR, et al. Computed to-mography scanning with image reconstruction in evaluation of distal radius fractures. J Hand Surg Am 1994;19:720–7.

34. Del Piñal F, Klausmeyer M, Moraleda E, et al. Arthroscopic reduction of comminuted intra-articular distal radius fractures with diaphyseal-metaphyseal comminution. J Hand Surg Am 2014;39(5):835–43.

35. Ono H, Furuta K, Fujitani R, et al. Distal radius fracture arthroscopic intraarticular displacement measurement after open reduction and internal fixation from a volar approach. J Orthop Sci 2010;15(4):502–8.

36. Del Piñal F, Clune J. Arthroscopic management of intra-articular malunion in fractures of the distal radius. Hand Clin 2017;33(4):669–75.

37. Smeraglia F, Del Buono A, Maffulli N. Wrist arthroscopy in the management of articular distal radius fractures. Br Med Bull 2016;119(1):157–65.

38. Saab M, Wunenburger PE, Guerre E, et al. Does arthroscopic assistance improve reduction in distal articular radius fracture? A retrospective comparative study using a blind CT assessment. Eur J Orthop Surg Traumatol 2019;29(2):405–11.

39. Yamazaki H, Uchiyama S, Komatsu M, et al. Arthroscopic assistance does not improve the functional or radiographic outcome of unstable intra-articular distal radial fractures treated with a volar locking plate: a randomised controlled trial. Bone Joint J 2015;97-B(7):957–62.

40. Ruch DS, Vallee J, Poehling GG, et al. Arthroscopic reduction versus fluoroscopic reduction in the management of intra-articular distal radius fractures. Arthroscopy 2004;20(3):225–30.

41. Abe Y, Fujii K. Arthroscopic-assisted reduction of intra-articular distal radius fracture. Hand Clin 2017;33(4):659–68.

42. Leclercq C, Mathoulin C, The members of EWAS. Complications of wrist arthroscopy: a multi-center study based on 10,107 arthroscopies. J Wrist Surg 2016;5(4):320–6.

43. Ahsan ZS, Yao J. Complications of wrist and hand arthroscopy. Hand Clin 2017;33(4):831–8.

44. Herzberg G. Intra-articular fracture of the distal radius: arthroscopic- assisted reduction. J Hand Surg Am 2010;35:1517–9.

Distal Radius Fracture and the Distal Radioulnar Joint

Christina Nypaver, MD[a],*, David J. Bozentka, MD[b]

KEYWORDS

- Distal radioulnar joint (DRUJ) • Triangular fibrocartilage complex • Ulnar styloid

KEY POINTS

- Injuries to the distal radioulnar joint are common in distal radius fractures.
- Knowledge of the bony and soft tissue anatomy and their contribution to congruency and stability of the distal radioulnar joint is critical to understanding injury patterns and their treatment options.
- Treatment goals in the acute setting should be to prevent future instability or incongruency of the distal radioulnar joint.
- Treatment goals in the chronic setting should be to restore stability and congruency of the distal radioulnar joint to allow for painless, full (or improved) motion of the wrist and forearm.
- Treatment in the chronic setting can be challenging.

INTRODUCTION

It is common knowledge that injury to the distal radioulnar joint (DRUJ) occurs frequently in the setting of a distal radius fracture. Failure to recognize and appropriately treat these concomitant injuries can lead to residual wrist disability and has been associated with worse functional outcomes.[1–7]

The DRUJ is a complex anatomic unit providing an articular link between the distal radius and ulna. It is composed of both bony and soft tissue structures that, along with the proximal radioulnar joint, allow for rotation (pronation/supination) of the forearm. It is critical that the hand surgeon understands the anatomy of the DRUJ when considering how injury in the setting of a distal radius fracture may alter its biomechanics. These alterations can lead to instability and incongruency, which can cause ulnar-sided wrist pain, limitations in range of motion, and the development of arthritis and ulnar impaction syndrome, which can ultimately affect function and quality of life.[1,6–12]

CONSIDERATIONS: ANATOMY

Review of Bony Distal Radioulnar Joint Anatomy

- The ulna is the stable unit of the forearm and its distal head includes an articular seat—a pivot point around which the radius rotates by means of its sigmoid notch.
- The radius of curvature of the sigmoid notch is greater than that of the ulnar seat and is concave and shallow, which allows the radius to rotate between 150° and 180° (**Fig. 1**).[13–16]
- The dorsal and volar rims or lips of the sigmoid notch contribute to joint stability; however, the bony anatomy is variable and inherently unstable. Thus, the soft tissue structures of the DRUJ are critical for stabilization.[14,16–18]
- The ulnar head also has a U-shaped pole or dome, which articulates with the triangular fibrocartilage complex (TFCC), the most important soft tissue stabilizer of the DRUJ.[5,15]
- The ulnar styloid is a bony projection that continues distally from the dome of the ulna; at its

[a] Department of Orthopaedic Surgery, University of Pennsylvania, 3737 Market Street, Philadelphia, PA 19104, USA; [b] Department of Orthopaedic Surgery, University of Pennsylvania, Penn Presbyterian Medical Center, 3737 Market Street, Philadelphia, PA 19104, USA
* Corresponding author.
E-mail address: Christina.Nypaver@pennmedicine.upenn.edu

Hand Clin 37 (2021) 293–307
https://doi.org/10.1016/j.hcl.2021.02.011
0749-0712/21/© 2021 Elsevier Inc. All rights reserved.

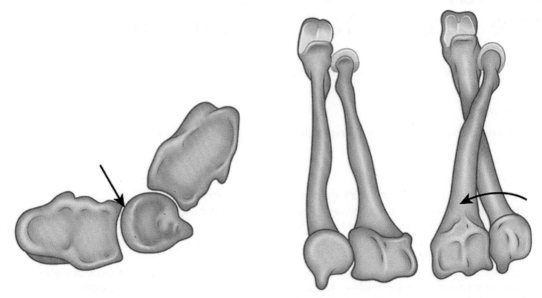

Fig. 1. Cross-sectional view of the DRUJ is shown on the left illustrating the difference in the radius of curvature between the radial sigmoid notch and the ulnar articular seat. The radius and the ulna on the right demonstrate the rotation of the 2 bones—the radius around the ulna—to allow for pronation and supination of the forearm and wrist.

base is a shallow concavity known as the fovea, which serves as a critical area for soft tissue attachment.[17]

- The distal ulna and its length relative to the distal radius varies among individuals, which is known as ulnar variance—an ulna longer than the radius is known as plus or positive variance, whereas an ulna shorter than the radius is known as minus or negative variance.[17]
  - Load transmissions at the ulnocarpal joint increase with positive variance, which also increases the likelihood of ulnar impaction or ulnocarpal abutment syndrome, where the distal ulna pathologically impacts or abuts the carpus.[15,19]
  - Ulnar variance can be measured on a standard posteroanterior view radiograph with the wrist in neutral.[20]
    - A line is drawn through the sclerotic line of the distal radius perpendicular to its longitudinal axis, and the variance is the distance between this line and the distal rim of the ulnar dome (**Fig. 2**).[21]

Review of Soft Tissue Distal Radioulnar Joint Anatomy

- The TFCC is composed of fibrocartilaginous and ligamentous structures that support the DRUJ and ulnocarpal articulations.[17,22]

- The dorsal and palmar radioulnar ligaments of the TFCC are essential for DRUJ stabilization.[17,22]
  - They originate from the dorsal and palmar margins of the sigmoid notch and divide in the coronal plane into superficial (distal) and deep (proximal) limbs.
  - The superficial limbs attach to the base and midportion of the ulnar styloid, whereas the deep limbs (also known as the *ligamentum subcruetum*) attach at the fovea (**Fig. 3**).[14,16,23]
  - The deep limbs are oriented in an obtuse fashion and use a pulling, tethering mechanism to confer profound stability to the DRUJ—the location of their anatomic insertion becomes clinically important when considering injury to the DRUJ in the setting of a distal radius fracture, particularly ulnar styloid fractures.[16,17]
  - The major constraint of dorsal translation of the distal ulna (relative to the radius) is the palmar radioulnar ligament, whereas the dorsal radioulnar ligament prevents palmar translation.[24,25]
- The triangular fibrocartilage proper (or articular disk) of the TFCC serves as an articular surface to absorb compressive loads from the carpus.[15,16]
- Other soft tissue stabilizers of the DRUJ include the pronator quadratus, the extensor

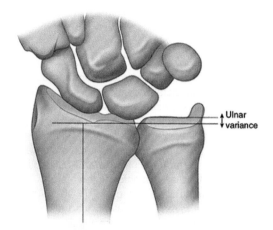

Fig. 2. Cartoon illustration of an anteroposterior (AP) view radiograph of the wrist and measurement of ulnar variance.

carpi ulnaris tendon, the DRUJ capsule, and the interosseous membrane, particularly the distal oblique bundle of the distal interosseous membrane, which is invariably present in the population.[5,13,14,16,17,25–30]

BACKGROUND

Approximately 2% to 37% of patients with distal radius fractures have DRUJ instability after their fracture has healed, and about two-thirds of these patients become symptomatic in the form of reduced range of motion and ulnar-sided wrist pain.[6,7,9,12,31] Injury to the DRUJ can take the form of bony injury, soft tissue injury, or a combination of both.[1] Predicting whether these injuries lead to clinically relevant or symptomatic DRUJ instability or incongruency continues to be evaluated in the literature.

CLINICAL RELEVANCE AND INCIDENCE OF DISTAL RADIOULNAR JOINT INJURIES
Distal Radius Fracture Deformity

Numerous studies have evaluated the impact of distal radius fracture characteristics and their role

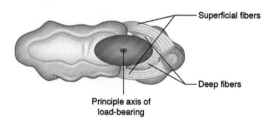

Fig. 3. Cross-sectional view of the DRUJ illustrating the deep and superficial palmar and dorsal radioulnar fibers of the TFCC and their respective anatomic origin and insertion sites.

in causing DRUJ instability or incongruency. Nakamura and colleagues[32] showed that radial translation and loss of radial inclination were significant predictors for a foveal avulsion of the radioulnar ligaments of the TFCC. Dy and colleagues[26] demonstrated that a coronal shift of 2 mm increased the dorsal–volar DRUJ displacement in cadaveric specimens with a distinct distal oblique bundle of the interosseous membrane. Other investigators have shown evidence of DRUJ incongruency or increased incidence of TFCC tears with volar or dorsal angulation of the distal radius, occurring in as little as 10° of angulation, and certainly with 20° of angulation.[14,33–38] Radial shortening is also associated with an increased risk for issues with the DRUJ.[34,39]

Logically, the correction of these deformities has the potential to restore stability of the DRUJ whereas persistent deformity in the form of a malunion can create alterations in DRUJ biomechanics and loss of tension of the stabilizing soft tissue structures.[9,28,36,40,41]

Intra-articular Extension (Sigmoid Notch)

Distal radius fractures with intra-articular extension into the sigmoid notch occur in about 55% of dorsally angulated intra-articular fractures, which may be more readily identifiable on computed tomography (CT) scans (**Fig. 4**).[42–44]

The obvious concern with intra-articular extension of any fracture is anatomic incongruency of the articular surface which can ultimately lead to degenerative changes and arthritis. Although 2 mm of intra-articular step-off for distal radius fractures has been widely accepted as the cutoff after which radiographic arthritis will almost certainly occur,[45] the majority of this research involves intra-articular extension into the radiocarpal joint, and not into the DRUJ.

Vitale and colleagues[46] evaluated patients with fracture extension into the sigmoid notch and found that these patients, when operatively treated, did not have a greater prevalence of DRUJ arthritis and that only fractures with a coronal step-off of greater than 1 mm had higher levels of upper extremity dysfunction according to Disabilities of the Arm, Shoulder, and Hand scoring. It, therefore, seems reasonable to apply the radiocarpal cutoff to the articular step-off involving the sigmoid notch.[47]

Intra-articular extension may also play a role in the development of DRUJ instability. Bombaci and colleagues[48] found that, when a fracture line extended into the sigmoid notch in conjunction with an associated ulnar styloid fracture, there was a greater incidence of an associated TFCC lesion than with other distal radius fracture types. A displaced fracture of the volar or dorsal rim of the sigmoid notch may lead to loss of the bony stability provided by the articulation resulting in DRUJ instability.

Ulnar Styloid Fractures

Associated ulnar styloid fractures are very common with distal radius fractures (≥50%).[4,16,34,39,49] Ulnar styloid fractures that occur at the base (basistyloid) have been more concerning for DRUJ instability, because the fragment includes the fovea, which signifies possible disruption of the insertion of the deep radioulnar fibers of the TFCC (**Fig. 5**).[4,5,50] Similarly, ulnar styloid fracture displacement of more than 2 mm has been reported to be associated with DRUJ instability.[4,50]

A number of studies have shown, however, that in operatively treated distal radius fractures without identifiable evidence of DRUJ instability, the presence of an ulnar styloid fracture does not affect functional outcomes, regardless of fracture displacement or location.[39,51–55] Possible explanations are that ulnar styloid fractures show less displacement after fixation of a distal radius fracture[39] or that there are other soft tissue stabilizers of the DRUJ that remain intact and maintain DRUJ stability and congruency.[56]

   Although some investigators argue that ulnar styloid nonunion is linked to instability of the DRUJ and "less favorable" outcomes,[45,57] other researchers have demonstrated that it is not associated with pain, instability, or diminished function after operatively treated distal radius fractures.[39,53,55,58]

Tears of the Triangular Fibrocartilage Complex

Tears of the TFCC are the most common associated injury with distal radius fractures, occurring in up to 84% of fractures.[1,9] Many investigators have evaluated the link between TFCC tears and DRUJ instability, particularly peripheral TFCC tears, which is the most common location for tears in distal radius fractures.[2] Kwon and colleagues[8] determined that all patients in their study who had DRUJ instability had deep TFCC avulsion tears from the fovea of the ulnar head or the sigmoid notch. These findings are similar to those from Lindau and colleagues,[2] who found that 10 of 11 patients with complete, arthroscopically confirmed peripheral TFCC tears had DRUJ instability at follow-up evaluation. In addition, Hermansdorfer and Kleinman[59] reported that patients with ulnar-sided wrist pain and subjective DRUJ laxity who also had peripheral TFCC avulsion tears from the ulnar fovea.

   Other investigators argue that the peripheral portion of the TFCC is well-vascularized[60] and,

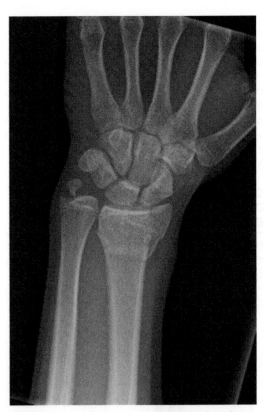

Fig. 5. Anteroposterior view radiograph of a left wrist demonstrating a basistyloid ulnar fracture in the setting of a distal radius fracture.

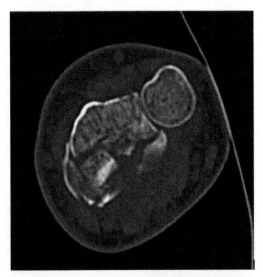

Fig. 4. Axial CT view of the DRUJ demonstrating an intra-articular distal radius fracture extending into the sigmoid notch.

therefore, has good healing potential as long as the ligaments are approximated and the patient is immobilized for a period of time to allow healing.[39] It should be noted that the vascular supply of the peripheral articular disk does decrease with age.[61]

ASSESSMENT, EVALUATION, AND IMAGING (ACUTE)

- A good history and physical examination is a must upon initial presentation.
  - Open wounds may indicate a higher energy mechanism and therefore an increased likelihood for DRUJ injury.[8]
- A crucial step in evaluating for an injury of the DRUJ is obtaining plain radiographs of the wrist with adequate views including a true lateral radiograph[32] and consideration of a CT scan if there is concern for intra-articular involvement.
- Imaging should permit evaluation of distal radius and distal ulna fracture characteristics that may be associated with an injury to the DRUJ (see Tears of the Triangular Fibrocartilage Complex and **Fig. 6**).
- Imaging can also allow for the identification of positive ulnar variance, widening of the DRUJ, or subluxation/dislocation of the ulna relative to the radius.
  - Positive ulnar variance of 6 mm or more and widening of the DRUJ by even 1 mm can increase the risk for DRUJ instability.[8,31,62,63]
- Tears of the TFCC can be diagnosed either by MRI or arthroscopically, which is the standard.

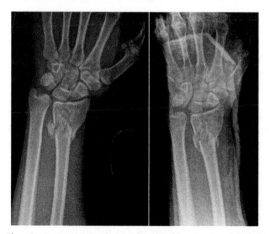

Fig. 6. Anteroposterior radiographic views of a left intra-articular distal radius fracture before (*left*) and after (*right*) closed reduction. There is a persistent widening of the DRUJ and new positive ulnar variance, concerning for an injury to the DRUJ.

- There is insufficient evidence to support obtaining MRIs for all acute, distal radius fractures.
- A TFCC tear that requires intervention in the acute setting is usually addressed intraoperatively.

Using these clues can assist the hand surgeon by raising their suspicion for a possible injury to the DRUJ. Most investigators would agree, however, that based on the literature discussed elsewhere in this article, a clinical assessment of the DRUJ should occur after anatomic reduction of the distal radius because this step, in and of itself, can restore stability and congruency to the DRUJ.[64] Most would also agree that this clinical assessment should be compared with the contralateral side because there can be ligamentous variability between patients.

Classification of Distal Radioulnar Joint Injuries (Acute)

The Fernandez classification can be a useful tool that defines the various combinations of injuries to the DRUJ in distal radius fractures and also guides treatment.[1] The treatment of DRUJ injuries consists of either early mobilization, closed treatment and immobilization with a cast with or without radioulnar pinning, or open versus arthroscopic treatment.

Injures are classified as type I, II, or III, which rely on the presence or absence of stability and the need for surgical intervention with increasing instability. Stability depends on the integrity of the sigmoid notch and the dorsal and volar radioulnar ligaments of the TFCC, and their insertion site on the fovea.

Type I injuries are stable, meaning there is articular congruity and the radioulnar ligaments are intact or minimally disrupted (ie, distal ulnar styloid "tip" fracture).[5] These injuries can be treated conservatively. Type II injuries are unstable despite an adequate reduction of the distal radius (could occur in large tears of the TFCC or *basistyloid* ulnar fracture), which do require surgical intervention. Type III injuries have the potential to be unstable and include disruption of the joint surface at the sigmoid notch or the ulnar head. These injuries require reduction and stabilization.

APPROACH FOR TREATMENT (ACUTE)

Before addressing the DRUJ, attention must first be directed toward the management of the distal radius fracture. As discussed in previous articles, displaced or angulated distal radius fractures should be close reduced and fractures that meet operative criteria should be treated surgically to restore length, alignment, and anatomic reduction of the articular surface, including fracture extension into the sigmoid notch.

Once satisfied with this reduction and/or fixation, the DRUJ should be examined radiographically—looking for persistent DRUJ widening, ulnar head subluxation relative to the radius, ulnar styloid fracture displacement, and so on—and clinically. Ideally, the contralateral, unaffected DRUJ and its stability are examined before the procedure.

Radioulnar stability can be examined clinically by a manual "shuck" test of the ulna, where the examiner rests the patient's upper extremity on the table with the elbow flexed and stabilizes the radius and wrist with one hand, while using their contralateral thumb and index finger to attempt to translate the ulnar head dorsal and palmar (mimicking a "piano key") within the sigmoid notch (**Fig. 7**).[5,16] Instability can be identified by a loss of a firm end point to translation or increased translation relative to the uninjured wrist. The test should be performed in neutral, pronation, and supination

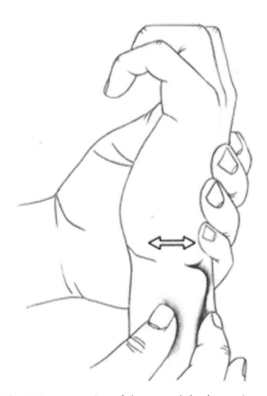

Fig. 7. Demonstration of the manual shuck examination maneuver. (*From* Kim JP, Park MJ. Assessment of Distal Radioulnar Joint Instability After Distal Radius Fracture: Comparison of Computed Tomography and Clinical Examination Results. *J Hand Surg Am.* 2008;33(9): 1486-1492.)

to ensure global stability and also to ensure that there are no blocks to forearm rotation. Although most surgeons usually do perform some variance of the shuck maneuver, a standard examination to detect instability has not been determined, and there is frequent interobserver reliability.[65] If there is no instability or blocks to motion, then no further intervention is required, even in the presence of an ulnar styloid fracture.[39]

If DRUJ instability or loss of motion is present, distal radius fracture reduction and hardware position should always be rechecked, first, and addressed if necessary. If the DRUJ continues to be unstable in some positions but stable in others, the patient should be immobilized in the position of stability, which is usually supination.[66] Immobilization can take the form of a splint followed by cast versus radioulnar Kirschner wire (K-wire) pinning of the DRUJ for 4 to 6 weeks. These pins are usually placed just proximal to the joint and include all 4 cortices of the radius and the ulna.

If the DRUJ is globally unstable and there is an ulnar styloid fracture (particularly a basistyloid location), the fracture should be addressed and fixed. The styloid fragment is reduced and can be fixed using nonabsorbable suture, a tension band construct, compression or cannulated headless screws, or an ulnar pin plate—all of which have been described (**Fig. 8**). Others have demonstrated that fixed outrigger external fixation can be an effective treatment option if the ulnar styloid can be reduced in maintained in supination.[67] The choice of fixation is dictated by the size of the fragment and surgeon preference.

It should be noted that ulnar-sided hardware can become symptomatic, particularly if the hardware irritates the extensor carpi ulnaris tendon, and may require subsequent removal. Immobilization duration should be dictated by satisfaction with stability of the reduction, that is, DRUJ stability should be re-examined after ulnar styloid fixation and can be combined with radioulnar pinning.

If the DRUJ is globally unstable and there is no ulnar styloid fracture or it is unstable despite good fixation of the ulnar styloid fracture, it should be assumed that there is disruption of the deep radioulnar fibers of the TFCC on their insertion at the fovea, and open or arthroscopic repair is indicated, usually in addition to radioulnar pinning[67–69] (see Jeffrey Yao and Nathaniel Fogel's article, "Arthroscopy in Distal Radius Fractures: Indications and When to Do It," in this issue). A tear of the deep radioulnar ligaments can be diagnosed arthroscopically, indirectly by loss of the "trampoline sign" and the presence of a positive hook test.[1,59,69] Central tears can be debrided,

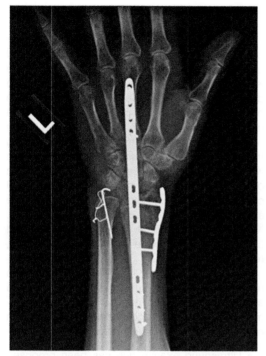

Fig. 8. Anteroposterior view radiograph of a left wrist demonstrating fixation of an ulnar styloid fracture using pinning with a tension band construct in the setting of an operatively treated distal radius fracture

radial avulsion tears can be repaired with a K-wire, and peripheral ulnar tears can be repaired with suture.[1] Patients should be immobilized anywhere from 4 to 8 weeks to allow the TFCC to heal. Sammer and Chung[47] presented a simplified algorithm to summarize treatment decision-making when there is presence of acute DRUJ instability (**Fig. 9**).

ASSESSMENT, EVALUATION, AND IMAGING (CHRONIC)

Issues related to the DRUJ after conservative or surgical treatment of a distal radius fractures can pose a unique challenge to the hand surgeon. These issues can generally be divided into 3 problems: (1) incongruency (which can lead to symptomatic arthritis), (2) positive ulnar variance (which can lead to symptomatic ulnar impaction/ulnocarpal abutment syndrome), and (3) instability. Even when these conditions are present, it is challenging to predict who will become symptomatic. Instability, for example, when present, may not necessarily correlate to long-term outcomes.[70]

- Patients presenting with wrist-related complaints after a distal radius fracture should undergo a comprehensive history and physical examination.
- The examiner should identify subtle deformities, localization and characteristics of pain, and any loss of range of motion—and compare these findings with the normal, contralateral side.
- Patients may present with a prominent or depressed ulnar head, loss of forearm pronation/supination, pain, and "clunking" with pronation/supination, or ulnar-sided wrist pain.
  - Clunking may represent reduction of a subluxating ulnar head back into the sigmoid notch.
  - Tenderness at the fovea could represent a TFCC tear.[71]
  - Extensor carpi ulnaris tendonitis also presents as ulnar-sided wrist pain with clicking and snapping of the tendon and should be included in the differential diagnosis.[72,73]

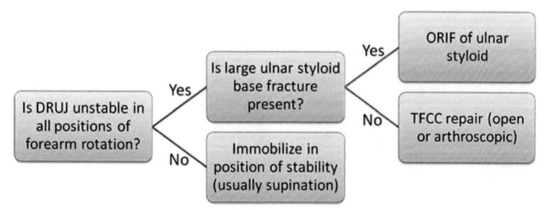

Fig. 9. Treatment algorithm for acute DRUJ instability in the setting of a distal radius fracture. (*From* Sammer DM, Chung KC. Management of the Distal Radioulnar Joint and Ulnar Styloid Fracture. *Hand Clin.* 2012;28(2): 199-206.)

- The manual shuck test should be performed in a similar fashion to specifically evaluate for radioulnar instability.
  - Pain can also be elicited during the maneuver because the patient will be awake.
- Plain view radiographs should be obtained first before other imaging modalities, because they can reveal pertinent and sometimes obvious clues about the etiology of a patient's complaints.
- The quality of the reduction of the distal radius in all planes should be critically analyzed.
  - A malunion should be identified as well as any hardware complications (loosening hardware, intra-articular penetration, etc) if the fracture was treated operatively (**Fig. 10**).
- Radiographs can also reveal persistent DRUJ widening, early signs of DRUJ arthritis, a displaced basistyloid ulnar fracture, or palmar or dorsal ulnar head subluxation seen on the lateral view.
  - Distances of 6 mm or more between the dorsal cortices of the distal radius and ulna should raise suspicion for DRUJ instability.[74]
- Ulnar variance can be measured and be compared with preoperative radiographs, if possible.
- CT scans can be useful for additional, detailed evaluation of a possible deformity causing a malunion,[75] subtle hardware complications, or persistent displacement of a fracture line extending into the sigmoid notch.[43]

CT scans have been evaluated for their capability to diagnose DRUJ instability. In this scenario, both wrists are imaged in neutral, pronated, and supinated positions.[72] There have been a number of proposed measurement methods, including the use of dorsal and palmar radioulnar lines,[76] the radioulnar ratio,[77] and via epicenter and congruency calculations.[72]

Lo and colleagues[77] presented the radioulnar ratio, which was found to be both reliable and practical in a clinical setting. A concentric circle is placed within the ulnar head and expanded to determine its center. A line is then drawn in the palmar–dorsal plane connecting the respective rims of the sigmoid notch. Finally, a line is drawn perpendicular to the previous line, intersecting the center of the ulnar head. The distance between where these 2 lines intersect and the volar margin of the sigmoid notch is then measured, and compared with the distance of the length of the sigmoid notch in the form of a ratio (**Fig. 11**). Normal ratios in neutral rotation, pronation, and supination were noted to be 0.50, 0.60, and 0.37, respectively.

These CT evaluations for DRUJ instability have received criticism, because they do not seem to accurately measure dynamic instability (ie, ligamentous injuries) and do not correlate well with physical examination stress tests.[78]

- Ultrasound examination has been proposed as an inexpensive, noninvasive study to evaluate for DRUJ instability, particularly dynamic instability.[79]
  - Physiologic translation of the DRUJ, however, has not been well-defined.
  - In neutral rotation, physiologic translation was determined to be 8 to 9 mm in cadaveric studies; however, some argue this is an overestimation when comparing with in vivo studies.[80–82]
- MRI or arthroscopy can detect TFCC tears as well as carpal changes in the presence of ulnar abutment syndrome.

Ultimately, diagnosing DRUJ instability (by examination or via imaging), and whether this is the

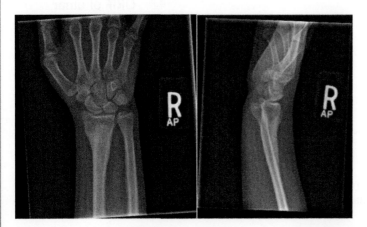

Fig. 10. Anteroposterior and lateral radiographic views of a right wrist demonstrating a healed, malunited distal radius fracture with widening of the DRUJ and volar subluxation of the ulna relative to the distal radius.

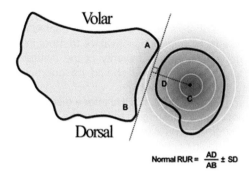

Normal RUR = $\frac{AD}{AB} \pm SD$

Fig. 11. The radioulnar (RUR) method for assessing DRUJ instability on an axial CT image. (Drawn by Rebecca Zhou.)

reason why a patient is symptomatic, can be difficult.

Classification of Distal Radioulnar Joint Injuries (Chronic)

Although not necessarily always related to a downstream effect of a distal radius fracture, Bowers and Zelouf[83] characterized chronic DRUJ disorders according to the presence of either (1) chronic joint disruption (instability), (2) ulnocarpal impingement, or (3) arthritis, and described treatment options for all 3 categories.

Chronic DRUJ instability owing to TFCC tears are recommended to be debrided arthroscopically, repaired, or reconstructed, whereas instability owing to bony injury should be addressed in the form of a corrective osteotomy or arthroplasty. In some cases, both ligamentous and bony injury may be present. Ulnocarpal impaction is treated with an ulnar shortening procedure. Arthritis is treated with various joint replacement and resection arthroplasty procedures, as well as arthrodesis procedures.

APPROACH FOR TREATMENT (CHRONIC)

Treatment should be aimed at the underlying etiology, which may not always be isolated, but rather a combination of issues. A treatment algorithm cannot as easily be developed. The goals of treatment should be to restore sigmoid notch congruency, correct any clinically relevant ulnar variance, and reestablish DRUJ stability to alleviate pain and improve range of motion.

The nonoperative management of symptomatic issues related to the DRUJ typically does provide long lasting relief. Immobilizing the wrist in the position of stability or strengthening the DRUJ stabilizers can be reasonable treatment options for low-demand patients.[84]

Malunion of the distal radius can cause structural incongruency of the DRUJ, which can lead to impingement and ulnocarpal abutment. Although beyond the scope of this article, the treatment of a distal radius malunion is usually addressed with an osteotomy with or without bone graft.[85–87] The distal radius is therefore realigned and the load distribution across the wrist is rebalanced. Osteotomies can also help to restore the bony anatomy and congruency of the sigmoid notch, and rebalance the ulnar variance if the distal radius was malunited in a shortened position compared with the ulna.[88,89]

In the absence of distal radius malunion, a symptomatic nonunion of the ulnar styloid can be treated with simple excision versus excision with TFCC stabilization to the remnant ulnar head via suture fixation with good results.[90] The fixation of a symptomatic ulnar styloid nonunion could be performed in a similar fashion as in an acute setting; however, attenuated soft tissues may preclude stabilization despite fixation.

If the DRUJ is congruent and there is positive ulnar variance causing symptomatic ulnar impaction or ulnocarpal abutment syndrome that cannot be corrected through a malunited distal radius osteotomy, then it is reasonable to proceed with an ulnar shortening osteotomy with a compression plate.[91–93]

Occasionally, the loss of forearm rotation could be caused by an isolated DRUJ capsule contracture. In the absence of other findings, a surgical release of the capsule could be indicated to restore motion.[13]

TFCC tears can cause pain or instability or both and, if present, should be addressed in a similar fashion as was described elsewhere in this article. A reduced distal radius and a competent sigmoid notch are prerequisites before these are addressed.

In some cases, TFCC tears can be irreparable and a reconstruction procedure to restore radioulnar ligament stability may be necessary. An extra-articular radioulnar tether,[94] an indirect sling/tenodesis tether,[73,95,96] and reconstruction of the radioulnar ligaments[97,98] have all been described. Although the extra-articular tether and the indirect sling/tenodesis tether can relieve pain, they have not been shown to restore physiologic DRUJ stability or biomechanics.[99]

Adams and Berger[100] described the anatomic reconstruction of the radioulnar ligaments using bone tunnels and a tendon graft (ie, palmaris longus), which has been shown to have an overall success rate of 86% at more than 5 years of follow-up (**Fig. 12**).[101]

It should be emphasized that any of these treatment procedures could be indicated in isolation

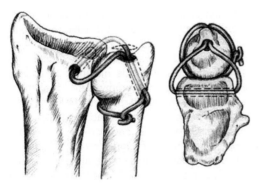

Fig. 12. Anteroposterior and axial views of the reconstruction of the palmar and dorsal radioulnar ligaments using a tendon graft. (Originally published in Adams BD, Berger RA. An anatomic reconstruction of the distal radioulnar ligaments for posttraumatic distal radioulnar joint instability. *J Hand Surg Am.* 2002;27(2):243-251.)

or in combination, depending on the etiology of clinical findings. For example, a distal radius malunion osteotomy may need to be combined with TFCC repair, and so on.

For patients with symptomatic DRUJ arthritis or who have failed these treatment options, salvage procedures may be the sole remaining options. These procedures might include a Sauve Kapandji arthrodesis of the DRUJ (useful for younger, active patients),[102–105] ulnar head resection arthroplasty (Darrach procedure),[106] or an ulnar prosthetic head replacement.

An additional salvage option is a hemiresection–interposition arthroplasty, which was first described by Bowers[107] in an attempt to combat the disadvantages of the Darrach procedure, which include loss of grip strength, loss of ulnar support of the carpus, and instability of the distal ulnar stump.[1] In this technique, the articular surface of the ulnar head is removed but retains the critical radioulnar attachments of the TFCC.

SUMMARY

Injuries to the DRUJ in the setting of a distal radius fracture are common. These injuries can be bony or soft tissue in nature, or a combination of these factors. A keen understanding of the anatomy of the DRUJ is critical. Hand surgeons should have a high index of clinical suspicion for any injury that might disrupt the congruency of the articular surfaces of the joint or the critical, stabilizing radioulnar ligaments of the TFCC and their insertion onto the ulnar fovea.

Achieving anatomic reduction of a distal radius fracture, whether acutely or chronically in the setting of a malunion, is a prerequisite and is the first step in treating a DRUJ injury. If instability persists in the acute setting, it should be treated in a stepwise fashion from less invasive to more invasive depending on the severity of the instability and any bony pathology should be addressed before soft tissue pathology.

Chronic injuries of the DRUJ after a distal radius fracture can be challenging to diagnose and treat. A thorough history, examination, and diagnostic workup should occur to determine the main underlying diagnoses and the best treatment options.

The goals of treatment in both the acute and chronic settings should emphasize congruency and stability of the DRUJ to allow for painless, functional range of motion of the forearm and wrist. As a last resort or in the setting of degenerative changes, salvage procedures may be necessary.

Overall, if detected, diagnosed, and managed appropriately, patients with distal radius fractures and concomitant injuries to the DRUJ can go on to have good functional outcomes and satisfaction.

CLINICS CARE POINTS

- Concomitant injuries to DRUJ with distal radius fractures are very common.
- Failure to address these injuries can lead to instability or incongruency of the joint, which can cause ulnar-sided wrist pain, limited range of motion of the wrist and forearm, and the development of arthritis and ulnar impaction syndrome.
- Understanding the bony and soft tissue anatomy of the DRUJ is critical.
  - The distal radius rotates around the distal ulna via the sigmoid notch.
  - The TFCC is the most important soft tissue stabilizer of the DRUJ, specifically the deep fibers of the dorsal and palmar radioulnar ligaments, which insert on the ulnar fovea.
- Injuries to the DRUJ can be bony, soft tissue, or a combination of both. Examples include the following.
  - Distal radius fracture deformity (leads to structural incongruency of the DRUJ).
  - Intra-articular extension into the sigmoid notch.
  - Ulnar styloid fractures (particularly basistyloid fractures, which include the foveal attachment site of the deep radioulnar ligaments).

○ TFCC tears.

Acute Setting

- High clinical index of suspicion for DRUJ injury with the known injury patterns.
- Radiographs should always be obtained; CT imaging may be indicated.
- A distal radius fracture should be anatomically reduced before evaluating for DRUJ instability and this evaluation should be compared with the normal, contralateral side.
- Persistent instability in an isolated position can be treated with immobilization (casting/radioulnar pinning) in the position of greatest stability.
- Persistent, global instability should be managed with fixation of the ulnar styloid fracture (if present) or repair of the deep radioulnar fibers of the TFCC (if an ulnar styloid fracture is not present or instability remains despite fixation of the ulnar styloid fracture).

Chronic Setting

- Issues related to the DRUJ after a distal radius fracture are usually related to incongruency (which can lead to arthritis), positive ulnar variance (which can lead to ulnar impaction syndrome), and/or instability.
- A thorough history, physical examination, and diagnostic workup should take place.
- Radiographs are mandatory; CT scans, MRI, and ultrasound imaging can provide useful supplemental information.
- Instability and whether this is the cause of patient symptoms can be challenging to diagnose.
- Distal radius fracture malunion should be addressed first with an osteotomy with or without bone graft (if present).
- In the absence of malunion and with a congruent DRUJ, a symptomatic ulnar styloid nonunion can be treated with excision with or without repair of the TFCC to the remnant ulnar base.
- Isolated positive ulnar variance causing ulnar impaction syndrome can be treated with an ulnar shortening osteotomy.
- Isolated, reparable TFCC tears should be fixed; nonreparable tears may require a reconstructive procedure.
- A combination of these procedures may be indicated.
- In the presence of arthritis or as a last resort, salvage procedures may be necessary.

DISCLOSURE

Dr C. Nypaver has nothing to disclose. Dr D.J. Bozentka has no funding source. Disclosures: Axogen principal investigator, speaker Medartis, Synthes.

REFERENCES

1. Geissler WB, Fernandez DL, Lamey DM. Distal radioulnar joint injuries associated with fractures of the distal radius. Clin Orthop Relat Res 1996;327:135–46.
2. Lindau T, Adlercreutz C, Aspenberg P. Peripheral tears of the triangular fibrocartilage complex cause distal radioulnar joint instability after distal radial fractures. J Hand Surg Am 2000;25(3):464–8.
3. Lindau T, Runnquist K, Aspenberg P. Patients with laxity of the distal radioulnar joint after distal radial fractures have impaired function, but no loss of strength. Acta Orthop Scand 2002;73(2):151–6.
4. May MM, Lawton JN, Blazar PE. Ulnar styloid fractures associated with distal radius fractures: incidence and implications for distal radioulnar joint instability. J Hand Surg Am 2002;27(6):965–71.
5. Distal radius fractures. In: Wolfe SW, Hotchkiss RN, Pederson WC, et al, editors. Green's operative hand surgery. 7th edition. Philadelphia: Elsevier; 2017. p. 516–07.
6. Oskarsson GV, Aaser P, Hjall A. Do we underestimate the predictive value of the ulnar styloid affection in Colles fractures? Arch Orthop Trauma Surg 1997;116(6–7):341–4.
7. Stoffelen D, De Smet L, Broos P. The importance of the distal radioulnar joint in distal radial fractures. J Hand Surg Br 1998;23(4):507–11.
8. Kwon BC, Seo BK, Im HJ, et al. Clinical and radiographic factors associated with distal radioulnar joint instability in distal radius fractures. Clin Orthop Relat Res 2012;470(11):3171–9.
9. Lindau T. Treatment of injuries to the ulnar side of the wrist occurring with distal radial fractures. Hand Clin 2005;21(3):417–25.
10. Ishikawa JI, Iwasaki N, Minami A. Influence of distal radioulnar joint subluxation on restricted forearm rotation after distal radius fracture. J Hand Surg Am 2005;30(6):1178–84.
11. Drobner WS, Hausman MR. The distal radioulnar joint. Hand Clin 1992;8(4):631–44.
12. Tsukazaki T, Iwasaki K. Ulnar wrist pain after Colles' fracture. 109 fractures followed for 4 years. Acta Orthop Scand 1993;64(4):462–4.
13. Kleinman WB, Graham TJ. The distal radioulnar joint capsule: clinical anatomy and role in posttraumatic limitation of forearm rotation. J Hand Surg Am 1998;23(4):588–99.
14. Ekenstam FA. Anatomy of the distal radioulnar joint. Clin Orthop Relat Res 1992;(275):14–8.

15. Linscheid RL. Biomechanics of the DRUJ. Clin Orthop Relat Res 1991;275:46–55.

16. Kleinman WB. Stability of the distal radioulnar joint: biomechanics, pathophysiology, physical diagnosis, and restoration of function what we have learned in 25 years. J Hand Surg Am 2007;32(7): 1086–106.

17. Adams BD, Leversedge FJ. Distal Radioulnar Joint. In: Wolfe SW, Hotchkiss RN, Pederson WC, et al, editors. Green's operative hand surgery. 7th edition. Philadelphia: Elsevier; 2017. p. 479–515.

18. Tolat AR, Stanley JK, Trail IA. A cadaveric study of the anatomy and stability of the distal radioulnar joint in the coronal and transverse planes. J Hand Surg Br 1996;21(5):587–94.

19. Palmer AK, Werner FW. Biomechanics of the distal radioulnar joint. Clin Orthop Relat Res 1984;187:26–35.

20. Yeh GL, Beredjiklian PK, Katz MA, et al. Effects of forearm rotation on the clinical evaluation of ulnar variance. J Hand Surg Am 2001;26(6):1042–6.

21. Steyers CM, Blair WF. Measuring ulnar variance: a comparison of techniques. J Hand Surg Am 1989; 14(4):607–12.

22. Palmer AK, Werner FW. The triangular fibrocartilage complex of the wrist–anatomy and function. J Hand Surg Am 1981;6(2):153–62.

23. Berger RA. The anatomy of the ligaments of the wrist and distal radioulnar joints. Clin Orthop Relat Res 2001;383:32–40.

24. Stuart PR, Berger RA, Linscheid RL, et al. The dorsopalmar stability of the distal radioulnar joint. J Hand Surg Am 2000;25(4):689–99.

25. Ward LD, Ambrose CG, Masson MV, et al. The role of the distal radioulnar ligaments, interosseous membrane, and joint capsule in distal radioulnar joint stability. J Hand Surg Am 2000;25(2):341–51.

26. Dy CJ, Jang E, Taylor SA, et al. The impact of coronal alignment on distal radioulnar joint stability following distal radius fracture. J Hand Surg Am 2014;39(7):1264–72.

27. Kitamura T, Moritomo H, Arimitsu S, et al. The biomechanical effect of the distal interosseous membrane on distal radioulnar joint stability: a preliminary anatomic study. J Hand Surg Am 2011; 36(10):1626–30.

28. Watanabe H, Berger RA, Berglund LJ, et al. Contribution of the interosseous membrane to distal radioulnar joint constraint. J Hand Surg Am 2005; 30(6):1164–71.

29. Noda K, Goto A, Murase T, et al. Interosseous membrane of the forearm: an anatomical study of ligament attachment locations. J Hand Surg Am 2009;34(3):415–22.

30. Ross M, Di Mascio L, Peters S, et al. Defining residual radial translation of distal radius fractures: a potential cause of distal radioulnar joint instability. J Wrist Surg 2014;03(02):158–60.

31. Fujitani R, Omokawa S, Akahane M, et al. Predictors of distal radioulnar joint instability in distal radius fractures. J Hand Surg Am 2011;36(12): 1919–25.

32. Nakamura T, Iwamoto T, Matsumura N, et al. Radiographic and arthroscopic assessment of DRUJ instability due to foveal avulsion of the radioulnar ligament in distal radius fractures. J Wrist Surg 2014;03(01):012–7.

33. Kihara H, Palmer AK, Werner FW, et al. The effect of dorsally angulated distal radius fractures on distal radioulnar joint congruency and forearm rotation. J Hand Surg Am 1996;21(1):40–7.

34. Richards RS, Bennett JD, Roth JH, et al. Arthroscopic diagnosis of intra-articular soft tissue injuries associated with distal radial fractures. J Hand Surg Am 1997;22(5):772–6.

35. Hirahara H, Neale PG, Lin Y Te, et al. Kinematic and torque-related effects of dorsally angulated distal radius fractures and the distal radial ulnar joint. J Hand Surg Am 2003;28(4):614–21.

36. Adams BD. Effects of radial deformity on distal radioulnar joint mechanics. J Hand Surg Am 1993; 18(3):492–8.

37. Nishiwaki M, Welsh MF, Gammon B, et al. Effect of volarly angulated distal radius fractures on forearm rotation and distal radioulnar joint kinematics. J Hand Surg Am 2015;40(11):2236–42.

38. Nishiwaki M, Welsh M, Gammon B, et al. Distal radioulnar joint kinematics in simulated dorsally angulated distal radius fractures. J Hand Surg Am 2014;39(4):656–63.

39. Kim JK, Koh Y Do, Do NH. Should an ulnar styloid fracture be fixed following volar plate fixation of a distal radial fracture? J Bone Joint Surg Am 2010; 92(1):1–6.

40. Crisco JJ, Moore DC, Marai GE, et al. Effects of distal radius malunion on distal radioulnar joint mechanics–an in vivo study. J Orthop Res 2007;25(4): 547–55.

41. Xing SG, Chen YR, Xie RG, et al. In vivo contact characteristics of distal radioulnar joint with malunited distal radius during wrist motion. J Hand Surg Am 2015;40(11):2243–8.

42. Tanabe K, Nakajima T, Sogo E, et al. Intra-articular fractures of the distal radius evaluated by computed tomography. J Hand Surg Am 2011; 36(11):1798–803.

43. Rozental TD, Bozentka DJ, Katz MA, et al. Evaluation of the sigmoid notch with computed tomography following intra-articular distal radius fracture. J Hand Surg Am 2001;26(2):244–51.

44. Heo YM, Roh J-Y, Kim S-B, et al. Evaluation of the sigmoid notch involvement in the intra-articular distal radius fractures: the efficacy of computed tomography compared with plain X-ray. Clin Orthop Surg 2012;4(1):83–90.

45. Knirk JL, Jupiter JB. Intra-articular fractures of the distal end of the radius in young adults. J Bone Joint Surg Am 1986;68(5):647–59.

46. Vitale M, Brogan D, Shin A, et al. Intra-articular fractures of the sigmoid notch of the distal radius: analysis of progression to distal radial ulnar joint arthritis and impact on upper extremity function in surgically treated fractures. J Wrist Surg 2016; 05(01):052–8.

47. Sammer DM, Chung KC. Management of the distal radioulnar joint and ulnar styloid fracture. Hand Clin 2012;28(2):199–206.

48. Bombaci H, Polat A, Deniz G, et al. The value of plain x-rays in predicting TFCC injury after distal radial fractures. J Hand Surg Eur 2008;33(3): 322–6.

49. Frykman G. Fracture of the distal radius including sequelae–shoulder-hand-finger syndrome, disturbance in the distal radio-ulnar joint and impairment of nerve function. A clinical and experimental study. Acta Orthop Scand 1967;(Suppl 108):3+.

50. Shaw JA, Bruno A, Paul EM. Ulnar styloid fixation in the treatment of posttraumatic instability of the radioulnar joint: a biomechanical study with clinical correlation. J Hand Surg Am 1990;15(5):712–20.

51. Sammer DM, Shah HM, Shauver MJ, et al. The effect of ulnar styloid fractures on patient-rated outcomes after volar locking plating of distal radius fractures. J Hand Surg Am 2009;34(9):1595–602.

52. Souer JS, Ring D, Matschke S, et al. Effect of an unrepaired fracture of the ulnar styloid base on outcome after plate-and-screw fixation of a distal radial fracture. J Bone Joint Surg Am 2009;91(4): 830–8.

53. Zenke Y, Sakai A, Oshige T, et al. The effect of an associated ulnar styloid fracture on the outcome after fixation of a fracture of the distal radius. J Bone Joint Surg Br 2009;91(1):102–7.

54. Kazemian GH, Bakhshi H, Lilley M, et al. DRUJ instability after distal radius fracture: a comparison between cases with and without ulnar styloid fracture. Int J Surg 2011;9(8):648–51.

55. Buijze GA, Ring D. Clinical impact of United versus nonunited fractures of the proximal half of the ulnar styloid following volar plate fixation of the distal radius. J Hand Surg Am 2010;35(2):223–7.

56. Jupiter JB. Commentary: the effect of ulnar styloid fractures on patient-rated outcomes after volar locking plating of distal radius fractures. J Hand Surg Am 2009;34(9):1603–4.

57. Wysocki RW, Ruch DS. Ulnar styloid fracture with distal radius fracture. J Hand Surg Am 2012; 37(3):568–9.

58. Wijffels M, Ring D. The influence of non-union of the ulnar styloid on pain, wrist function and instability after distal radius fracture. J Hand Microsurg 2016;03(01):11–4.

59. Hermansdorfer JD, Kleinman WB. Management of chronic peripheral tears of the triangular fibrocartilage complex. J Hand Surg Am 1991;16(2):340–6.

60. Bednar MS, Arnoczky SP, Weiland AJ. The microvasculature of the triangular fibrocartilage complex: its clinical significance. J Hand Surg Am 1991;16(6):1101–5.

61. Mikić ZD. Age changes in the triangular fibrocartilage of the wrist joint. J Anat 1978;126(Pt 2): 367–84.

62. Iida A, Omokawa S, Akahane M, et al. Distal radioulnar joint stress radiography for detecting radioulnar ligament injury. J Hand Surg Am 2012;37(5): 968–74.

63. Omokawa S, Iida A, Fujitani R, et al. Radiographic Predictors of DRUJ instability with distal radius fractures. J Wrist Surg 2014;03(01):002–6.

64. Liu J, Wu Z, Li S, et al. Should distal radioulnar joint be fixed following volar plate fixation of distal radius fracture with unstable distal radioulnar joint? Orthop Traumatol Surg Res 2014;100(6):599–603.

65. Moriya T, Aoki M, Iba K, et al. Effect of triangular ligament tears on distal radioulnar joint instability and evaluation of three clinical tests: a biomechanical study. J Hand Surg Eur 2009;34(2):219–23.

66. Trousdale RT, Amadio PC, Cooney WP, et al. Radioulnar dissociation. A review of twenty cases. J Bone Joint Surg Am 1992;74(10):1486–97.

67. Ruch DS, Lumsden BC, Papadonikolakis A. Distal radius fractures: a comparison of tension band wiring versus ulnar outrigger external fixation for the management of distal radioulnar instability. J Hand Surg Am 2005;30(5):969–77.

68. Böhringer G, Schädel-Höpfner M, Junge A, et al. Die arthroskopische Therapie frischer Discus articularis Verletzungen bei distalen Radiusfrakturen. Handchir Mikrochir Plast Chir 2001;33:245–51.

69. Ruch DS, Yang CC, Smith BP. Results of acute arthroscopically repaired triangular fibrocartilage complex injuries associated with intra-articular distal radius fractures. Arthroscopy 2003;19(5): 511–6.

70. Wijffels MME, Krijnen P, Schipper IB. Clinical DRUJ instability does not influence the long-term functional outcome of conservatively treated distal radius fractures. Eur J Trauma Emerg Surg 2017; 43(2):227–32.

71. Tay SC, Tomita K, Berger RA. The "ulnar fovea sign" for defining ulnar wrist pain: an analysis of sensitivity and specificity. J Hand Surg Am 2007; 32(4):438–44.

72. Wechsler RJ, Wehbe MA, Rifkin MD, et al. Computed tomography diagnosis of distal radioulnar subluxation. Skeletal Radiol 1987;16(1):1–5.

73. Breen TF, Jupiter JB. Extensor carpi ulnaris and flexor carpi ulnaris tenodesis of the unstable distal ulna. J Hand Surg Am 1989;14(4):612–7.

74. Nakamura R, Horii E, Imaeda T, et al. Distal radio-ulnar joint subluxation and dislocation diagnosed by standard roentgenography. Skeletal Radiol 1995;24(2):91–4.

75. Filer J, Smith A, Giddins G. Assessing distal radius malrotation following fracture using computed tomography. J Orthop Surg (Hong Kong) 2019; 27(3). 2309499019862872.

76. Mino DE, Palmer AK, Levinsohn EM. Radiography and computerized tomography in the diagnosis of incongruity of the distal radio-ulnar joint. A prospective study. J Bone Joint Surg Am 1985;67(2): 247–52.

77. Lo IK, MacDermid JC, Bennett JD, et al. The radioulnar ratio: a new method of quantifying distal radioulnar joint subluxation. J Hand Surg Am 2001; 26(2):236–43.

78. Kim JP, Park MJ. Assessment of distal radioulnar joint instability after distal radius fracture: comparison of computed tomography and clinical examination results. J Hand Surg Am 2008;33(9):1486–92.

79. Hess F, Farshad M, Sutter R, et al. A novel technique for detecting instability of the distal radioulnar joint in complete triangular fibrocartilage complex lesions. J Wrist Surg 2012;01(02):153–8.

80. Pirela-Cruz MA, Goll SR, Klug M, et al. Stress computed tomography analysis of the distal radioulnar joint: a diagnostic tool for determining translational motion. J Hand Surg Am 1991;16(1):75–82.

81. Pan C-C, Lin Y-M, Lee T-S, et al. Displacement of the distal radioulnar joint of clinically symptom-free patients. Clin Orthop Relat Res 2003;415:148–56.

82. Haugstvedt J-R, Berger RA, Berglund LJ, et al. An analysis of the constraint properties of the distal radioulnar ligament attachments to the ulna. J Hand Surg Am 2002;27(1):61–7.

83. Bowers W, Zelouf D. Treatment of chronic disorders of the distal radioulnar joint. In: LIchtman D, editor. The wrist and its disorders. 2nd edition. Philadelphia: WB Saunders; 1997.

84. Millard GM, Budoff JE, Paravic V, et al. Functional bracing for distal radioulnar joint instability. J Hand Surg Am 2002;27(6):972–7.

85. Fernandez DL. Correction of post-traumatic wrist deformity in adults by osteotomy, bone-grafting, and internal fixation. J Bone Joint Surg Am 1982; 64(8):1164–78.

86. Fernandez DL. Reconstructive procedures for malunion and traumatic arthritis. Orthop Clin North Am 1993;24(2):341–63.

87. af Ekenstam F, Hagert CG, Engkvist O, et al. Corrective osteotomy of malunited fractures of the distal end of the radius. Scand J Plast Reconstr Surg 1985;19(2):175–87.

88. Cooney WP 3rd, Dobyns JH, Linscheid RL. Complications of Colles' fractures. J Bone Joint Surg Am 1980;62(4):613–9.

89. Cheng C-Y, Chang C-H. Corrective osteotomy for intra-articular malunion of the sigmoid notch of the distal part of the radius: a case report. Hand Surg 2008;13(2):93–7.

90. Hauck RM, Skahen J 3rd, Palmer AK. Classification and treatment of ulnar styloid nonunion. J Hand Surg Am 1996;21(3):418–22.

91. Tränkle M, van Schoonhoven J, Krimmer H, et al. [Indication and results of ulna shortening osteotomy in ulnocarpal wrist joint pain]. Unfallchirurg 2000;103(3):197–202.

92. Srinivasan RC, Jain D, Richard MJ, et al. Isolated ulnar shortening osteotomy for the treatment of extra-articular distal radius malunion. J Hand Surg Am 2013;38(6):1106–10.

93. Chen NC, Wolfe SW. Ulna shortening osteotomy using a compression device. J Hand Surg Am 2003;28(1):88–93.

94. Fulkerson JP, Watson HK. Congenital anterior subluxation of the distal ulna. A case report. Clin Orthop Relat Res 1978;131:179–82.

95. Tsai TM, Stilwell JH. Repair of chronic subluxation of the distal radioulnar joint (ulnar dorsal) using flexor carpi ulnaris tendon. J Hand Surg Br 1984; 9(3):289–94.

96. Hui FC, Linscheid RL. Ulnotriquetral augmentation tenodesis: a reconstructive procedure for dorsal subluxation of the distal radioulnar joint. J Hand Surg Am 1982;7(3):230–6.

97. Adams BD. Anatomic Reconstruction of the Distal Radioulnar Ligaments for DRUJ Instability. Tech Hand Up Extrem Surg 2000;4(3):154–60.

98. Scheker LR, Belliappa PP, Acosta R, et al. Reconstruction of the dorsal ligament of the triangular fibrocartilage complex. J Hand Surg Br 1994;19(3): 310–8.

99. Petersen MS, Adams BD. Biomechanical evaluation of distal radioulnar reconstructions. J Hand Surg Am 1993;18(2):328–34.

100. Adams BD, Berger RA. An anatomic reconstruction of the distal radioulnar ligaments for posttraumatic distal radioulnar joint instability. J Hand Surg Am 2002;27(2):243–51.

101. Gillis JA, Soreide E, Khouri JS, et al. Outcomes of the Adams–Berger ligament reconstruction for the distal radioulnar joint instability in 95 consecutive cases. J Wrist Surg 2019;08(04):268–75.

102. Zilch H, Kauschke T. [Kapandji corrective operation of post-traumatic disorder of the distal radioulnar joint]. Unfallchirurg 1996;99(11):841–4.

103. Preisser P, Buck-Gramcko D, Hess J. [Distal radio-ulnar arthrodesis and Kapandji ulna segment resection in treatment of limited forearm rotation]. Handchir Mikrochir Plast Chir 1991; 23(5):255–61.

104. Mikkelsen SS, Lindblad BE, Larsen ER, et al. Sauvé-Kapandji operation for disorders of the

distal radioulnar joint after Colles' fracture. Good results in 12 patients followed for 1.5-4 years. Acta Orthop Scand 1997;68(1):64–6.

105. Kapandji IA. The Kapandji-Sauvé operation. Its techniques and indications in non rheumatoid diseases. Ann Chir Main 1986;5(3): 181–93.

106. Imbriglia JE, Matthews D. Treatment of chronic post-traumatic dorsal subluxation of the distal ulna by hemiresection-interposition arthroplasty. J Hand Surg Am 1993;18(5):899–907.

107. Bowers WH. Distal radioulnar joint arthroplasty: the hemiresection-interposition technique. J Hand Surg Am 1985;10(2):169–78.

Is Therapy Needed After Distal Radius Fracture Treatment, What Is the Evidence?

Paul Kooner, MD[a], Ruby Grewal, MD, MSc, FRCSC[b],*

KEYWORDS

- Distal radius fracture • Rehabilitation • Hand therapy

KEY POINTS

- Encouraging early ROM and return to routine activities of daily living is an essential component of recovery.
- A single instructional session with a home based program may be as effective as formal supervised therapy.
- Formal structured therapy may play a role in select high-risk patients.

BACKGROUND

Distal radius fractures (DRFs) are one of the most common orthopedic injuries sustained by the adult population.[1] These fractures are frequently the result of low-energy falls in the elderly population and high-energy trauma in younger adults. The goals of treatment are to restore anatomy and maintain optimal function of the wrist. Rehabilitation with exercise and other physical interventions are often used to help prevent complications and to facilitate recovery.

DRFs usually require 4 to 6 weeks to achieve bony union and 6 to 12 months to completely restore motion, strength, and function. Expected time to regain function varies and relates to injury severity and patient factors, dependent on their individual physical and recreational demands.[2–5] The goals of treatment are to maximize function (grip strength and range of motion [ROM]) and to minimize adverse events (stiffness, complex regional pain syndrome, tendon rupture, tendinitis).

The rehabilitation process often uses various health care professionals and resources. Although the orthopedic surgeon provides the definitive fracture management, physical and occupational therapists are often involved with the rehabilitation of these injuries. Many of these therapists are specialized in hand and upper limb function and they aid patients to achieve independence in their routine activities of daily living. However, recent evidence has shown that their role in facilitating patient recovery is unclear.[6,7] Current concerns regarding rehabilitation after DRFs are centered around a few basic questions: When should therapy be initiated and for how long? What modalities should be used? Is there an advantage to a formal supervised therapy program compared with a home program? Can therapy influence final outcomes?

As clinicians treating DRFs, we must endeavor to optimize recovery. The purpose of this article was to review the current evidence evaluating the role of rehabilitation and hand therapy after DRFs, to discuss the various therapeutic options used, and to compare their relative effectiveness. Last, we aimed to provide recommendations

---

[a] Orthopaedic Surgery PGY1, McGill University, 1650 Cedar Avenue, Montreal, Quebec H3G 1A4, Canada;
[b] Division of Orthopaedic Surgery, Roth|McFarlane Hand and Upper Limb Center, Western University, D0-217, St Joseph's Health Care, 268 Grosvenor Street, London, Ontario N6A 4V2, Canada
* Corresponding author.
E-mail address: rgrewa@uwo.ca

Hand Clin 37 (2021) 309–314
https://doi.org/10.1016/j.hcl.2021.02.012
0749-0712/21/© 2021 Elsevier Inc. All rights reserved.

based on the latest evidence for the role of rehabilitation after DRFs.

WHEN TO INITIATE THERAPY?

Initial therapy goals include pain management, edema management, and maintenance of ROM of the adjacent joints. More extensive rehabilitation usually begins once indicated by the treating surgeon. This may be dictated by fracture stability, choice of fixation, and extent of fracture union. Later treatment goals expand to address limited ROM, impaired dexterity, and reduced grip strength, with an aim to restore function, maximize outcomes, and minimize complications.

When to commence rehabilitation after DRF remains a controversial topic. Therapy may be initiated immediately after the injury is sustained and/or undertaken once the initial treatment period is over (ie, after the cast is removed). On receiving initial clinical treatment, patients are usually given instructions to carry out a set of standardized exercises independently.

A prospective randomized controlled trial with 81 participants evaluated an accelerated versus standard rehabilitation protocol for DRFs treated with volar locking plate fixation.[8] They compared the outcomes between an accelerated program (started at 2 weeks) versus usual rehabilitation (started at 6 weeks) after volar locking plate fixation. Both groups began with gentle active wrist ROM at 3 to 5 days postoperatively. At 2 weeks postoperatively, the accelerated group initiated wrist and forearm passive ROM and strengthening exercises, whereas the standard group commenced passive ROM and strengthening exercises at 6 weeks postoperatively. In the accelerated group, Disability of Arm Shoulder and Hand (DASH) scores showed a clinically and statistically significant advantage up to 8 weeks after surgery. They found that the differences in the postoperative ROM and DASH scores suggest an earlier return to function by patients who followed the accelerated protocol. Although, beyond 12 weeks there was little difference in outcomes between the 2 groups.

A similar randomized control trial (RCT) conducted by Lozano-Calderon and colleagues[9] examined 60 patients who mobilized the wrist joint at either 2 weeks or at 6 weeks after volar plate fixation. The primary outcome was the flexion-extension arc at 3 and 6 months. There were no significant differences between the early motion group and the late motion group with regard to the average flexion-extension arc of the wrist at either 3 or 6 months.[9] Secondary outcomes included grip strength, radiographic parameters, the modified Gartland and Werley Score, Mayo Wrist Score, and pain and DASH scores, all of which showed no significant differences between the 2 groups. This study concluded that initiation of wrist exercises at 6 weeks after volar plate fixation did not lead to decreased wrist motion when compared with the initiation of exercises at 2 weeks after surgery.

An accelerated rehabilitation protocol started as soon as 2 weeks postoperatively may optimize short-term functional outcomes; however, it did not influence final outcomes. The short-term functional advantages gained with an early rehabilitation program may be important for certain patient groups; for example, elderly patients whose functional independence depends on maximizing upper extremity function or individuals aiming to minimize time away from work or sport. Long-term data suggest these findings are equivocal between the 2 groups and clinicians must decide whether the short-term advantage is meaningful for their patients and initiate therapy accordingly.

HOME VERSUS SUPERVISED PROGRAMS

Hand therapy following DRFs is generally regarded as an important part of rehabilitation and recovery. Patients are routinely referred to a hand therapist and may receive treatment for extended periods; however, there is a paucity of literature examining the advantage of a supervised treatment program versus home exercise programs, and the subsequent influence on clinical outcomes after DRFs. Recent literature has examined the effectiveness of such treatment protocols and questioned the benefits of prolonged supervised therapy after DRF.

An RCT conducted by Wakefield and McQueen[6] studied the impact of physiotherapy on clinical outcomes after DRFs in 96 patients. Patient outcomes were compared between conventional physiotherapy and a home exercise regimen. Their results showed that there was no difference in hand function and grip strength between the 2 groups. Only wrist ROM in flexion and extension at 6 months' follow-up showed a significant advantage with therapy; however, there was no correlation between these results and the patient's functional scores. Overall quality of life was assessed using the Short Form-36 physical and mental scores, and conventional physiotherapy did not influence the well-being of these patients. The investigators concluded that the mode of delivery of physiotherapy had no proven effect on recovery after a DRF.

A systematic review compared the role of prescribed exercise in the management of DRF rehabilitation.[10] It examined any exercise therapy program, including trials in which patients received any form of supervised therapy, home exercises, or no intervention at all. There was insufficient evidence to support the effectiveness of either a home-based or supervised exercise regimen in 13 identified trials. The review also identified 3 studies in which home or supervised therapy was compared with no intervention at all.[11–13] The results of 2 studies showed no difference in functional or patient-reported outcomes.[11,12] The third study found a slight benefit of supervised therapy in patient-reported outcomes but no differences in functional outcomes.[13] However, this study was limited to 6 weeks of follow-up and may be insufficient to allow for therapy comparisons. These findings illustrate the limitations of such a review, as it cannot standardize a therapy protocol between studies, allowing for discrepancies in the types of intervention and duration of therapies compared.

A recent RCT conducted by Chung and colleagues[14] in 2019 explored the relationship between hand therapy and long-term outcomes after DRFs in older adults. This trial followed 268 patients who either underwent supervised physiotherapy sessions or those who only received home exercises. At 12 months there were no differences in patient-reported outcomes based on participation in a formal supervised therapy versus a home exercise program. There were no differences in functional outcomes except that patients who underwent supervised therapy were shown to recover greater grip strength. Interestingly, overall quality-of-life scores revealed that a shorter duration of therapy was attributable to greater function, ability to work, and satisfaction. The investigators concluded that encouraging patients to resume activities of daily living as soon as possible may be as effective as formal therapy in producing satisfactory clinical outcomes after DRFs.

Although the literature trends toward minimal benefit of supervised therapy, there are certain high-risk patients who are expected to have worse outcomes and there is a concern that these patients should be followed more closely. Patients with high levels of baseline pain and those with tendencies toward catastrophic thinking or underlying psychological conditions, such as anxiety or depression, have been associated with increased disability and pain after orthopedic trauma.[15–18] Guidelines by the British Society for Surgery of the Hand for best practice management after DRF recommend that patients who experience disproportionate levels of pain or have delayed functional recovery should be referred to hand therapy for further evaluation and treatment.[19] These high-risk patients may benefit from supervised therapy to provide the psychological support

necessary to optimize outcomes. Early identification of these patients after DRFs and appropriate follow-up with a guided rehabilitation program may help optimize functional outcomes in this subset population. However, further research in this area is warranted.

The results of these studies suggest there is limited benefit of a supervised rehabilitation regimen when compared with a home exercise program. Interestingly, having a patient return to routine activities of daily living as soon as possible after treatment was shown to have just as effective clinical and functional outcomes compared with those who received formalized therapy. In this regard, we suggest implementing a single instruction session and home-based exercise program while motivating patients to return to routine activities as soon as tolerated by the individual. However, certain high-risk subgroups may benefit from a supervised program. Further research in this area is needed.

PASSIVE MODALITIES

There are many interventions currently used in the rehabilitation of DRFs, including but not limited to, patient education regarding recovery, home and supervised mobility and strengthening exercises, continuous passive motion, pain management using transcutaneous electrical nerve stimulation, heat, massage, whirlpool, and wound care. Further therapeutic options include specific physiotherapy and occupational therapy with home assessment and social support options to help optimize the patient's recovery. As there are no standardized guidelines for the use of these modalities in recovery after DRFs, a wide range of protocols are implemented with no clear evidence supporting their use. In this section, we aim to provide the current evidence of the use of various treatment modalities used in recovery after DRFs.

During cast immobilization, therapists initiate ROM exercises in the digits with both passive and active mobilization. Through mobilization, therapists are able to prevent upper extremity stiffness in addition to reducing edema. At this stage, pain management is treated with hot/cold modalities and compressive wraps.[20,21] Once the immobilization period is over, which is typically between 2 and 6 weeks after treatment, a more aggressive therapy regimen is commenced. During this phase, the goals include decreasing pain and edema; improvement in ROM of the hand, wrist, and forearm; and improvement in functional abilities. A combination of resistance exercises, joint mobilization, and heat are all used to increase ROM and decrease pain.[22,23] Further modalities, such as static progressive splinting, electrotherapy, whirlpool therapy, ultrasound, and massage, are also found to be used during this phase.[24–27] The final phase involves strengthening exercises and functional training that are tailored to the patient to return to routine activities of daily living.

A Cochrane review published by Handoll and Elliot[28] examined the various rehabilitation interventions in adults with conservatively or surgically treated DRFs. This review included 26 trials encompassing more than 1200 participants and discussed the relative effectiveness of specific interventions used in the rehabilitation of DRFs. When implementing single-intervention techniques, including passive mobilization, ice, electrotherapy, whirlpool, or dynamic splinting, it did not add to the effectiveness of conventional therapy when compared with no intervention at all, although there was low-quality evidence supporting short-term benefit from the use of continuous passive movement after external fixation, intermittent pneumatic compression, and ultrasound therapy. Although many of these techniques are used by therapists within their rehabilitation protocols, to date there is limited research evaluating their relative effectiveness on outcomes. This thorough review illustrates the limited use of such therapies after DRFs and shows they do not influence overall outcomes. Furthermore, this review reveals the heterogeneity in the application of such modalities, as there are a wide range and combination of use of these treatments found in the literature. With no standardized protocols guiding the use of these passive modalities, and no clear benefit in functional or clinical outcomes, their use after DRFs are limited.

When comparing therapy provided by either an occupational therapist or a physiotherapist, there is minimal evidence to suggest one discipline is superior to the other.[11,29,30] There were no statistically significant differences reported between the 2 groups in functional scores, pain scores, grip strength, or ROM at various time intervals. It was found that more "symptomatic" patients with decreased ROM and pain were favored to undergo physiotherapy versus occupational therapy, possibly noting observed differences at baseline. However, long-term outcome measures and quality-of-life scales showed no difference in outcomes.

COMPLICATION MANAGEMENT

Although the preceding evidence trends toward a minimal benefit of hand therapy and rehabilitation protocols in DRF treatment, there are subsets of the population that may benefit from formal, supervised therapy. Patients with complications or those who are at risk of poor outcomes may need therapy to optimize outcomes. Complex regional pain syndrome (CRPS) is a well-documented complication of both operatively and nonoperatively managed DRFs. It is characterized by burning sensation or pain, swelling, and changes in color, temperature, and perspiration of the affected limb.[31] With an incidence ranging from 2% to 37% and no definitive treatment of this syndrome, a combination of psychiatric therapy, hand therapy, and pain management has been shown to produce the best recovery.[32–34] Passive and active ROM, splinting, contrast baths, mirror therapy, and oral medication are considered first-line treatment.[32] Treatment may vary based on the severity of symptoms. Although the cause of CRPS remains unclear, studies have linked underlying risk factors, such as psychiatric conditions, fibromyalgia, and rheumatoid arthritis, to its development.[35] Further understanding of psychosocial factors that contribute to complications or patient outcomes may play a role in therapy-based interventions.

The understanding of psychosocial factors has improved the surgeon's ability to predict fracture outcomes. Symonette and colleagues[36] examined the role of social support in patient-reported pain and disability 1 year after DRF. The Medical Outcomes Study Social Support Survey was administered prospectively to 291 subjects with DRFs. At 1 year after treatment, emotional and informational support was found to explain 4.7% of the variance in patient-reported pain and disability. This highlights the potential rehabilitative benefits of improved social support and may be useful in optimizing outcomes for individuals with minimal support.

Key Findings and Clinical Care Points

- The available evidence is insufficient to establish a definitive role for hand therapy after DRFs and further investigations are warranted.

- When comparing modalities of therapy, there are no differences in outcomes of patients receiving routine supervised hand therapy versus instructions for home-based exercises.

- Encouraging patients to resume activities of daily living as soon as possible may be as effective as formal therapy.

- Accelerated rehabilitation started during the immobilization period may produce increased short-term functional outcomes, but long-term data remain equivocal.

- Therapy is warranted for high-risk population groups specifically for those with complications such as CRPS and underlying psychosocial issues that may contribute to poor outcomes.

In summary, the role of a formalized hand therapy program in the management and recovery after DRFs is unclear. There is some evidence demonstrating that initiating early ROM exercises and urging patients to return to routine activities of daily living as soon as possible may be just as effective as formal therapy in producing favorable clinical outcomes. It is clear that extended supervised therapy does not impact outcomes, and a single instruction session with a home-based program produces similar results. Although most patients can expect excellent outcomes after just a single instruction session and a home-based exercise program, we feel that formal structured therapy has a role in select patients whose recovery is slow and may help optimize recovery in certain high-risk subgroups.

CLINICS CARE POINTS

- Most patients will benefit from a single instruction hand therapy session followed by a home-based exercise program.
- Initiating early ROM and strengthening exercises after definitive management may minimize time away from work or sport in the early postoperative period.
- Patients experiencing complications, certain high-risk groups, or those slow to recovery may benefit from formal supervised hand therapy.
- Further research is warranted for the role of passive modalities in hand therapy after DRFs.

DISCLOSURE

Dr P. Kooner and Dr R. Grewal have no disclosure to report.

REFERENCES

1. Chung KC, Spilson SV. The frequency and epidemiology of hand and forearm fractures in the United States. J Hand Surg Am 2001;26(5):908–15.
2. Singer BR, McLauchlan GJ, Robinson CM, et al. Epidemiology of fractures in 15,000 adults: the influence of age and gender. J Bone Joint Surg 1998; 80B:243–8.
3. Vogt MT, Cauley JA, Tomaino MM, et al. Distal radius fractures in older women: A 10-year follow-up study of descriptive characteristics and risk factors: The study of osteoporotic fractures. J Am Geriatr Soc 2001;50:97–103.
4. O'Neill TW, Cooper C, Finn JD, et al. Incidence of distal forearm fracture in British men and women. Osteoporos Int 2001;12(7):555–8.
5. Court-Brown CM, Caesar B. Epidemiology of adult fractures: A review. Injury 2006;37(8):691–7.
6. Wakefield AE, McQueen MM. The role of physiotherapy and clinical predictors of outcome after fracture of the distal radius. J Bone Joint Surg 2000;82-B:972–6.
7. Golden GN. Treatment and prognosis of Colles' fracture. Lancet 1963;1:511–5.
8. Brehmer JL, Husband JB. Accelerated rehabilitation compared with a standard protocol after distal radius fractures treated with volar open reduction and internal fixation. J Bone Joint Surg Am 2014; 96:1621–30.
9. Lozano-Calderon SA, Souer S, Mudgal C, et al. Wrist mobilization following volar plate fixation of fractures of the distal part of the radius. J Bone Joint Surg Am 2008;90:1297–304.
10. Bruder AM, Shields N, Dodd KJ, et al. Prescribed exercise programs may not be effective in reducing impairments and improving activity during upper limb fracture rehabilitation: a systematic review. J Physiother 2017;63:205–20.
11. Souer JS, Buijze G, Ring D. A prospective randomized controlled trial comparing occupational therapy with independent exercises after volar plate fixation of a fracture of the distal part of the radius. J Bone Joint Surg Am 2011;93:1761–6.
12. Valdes K, Naughton N, Burke CJ. Therapist-supervised hand therapy versus home therapy with therapist instruction following distal radius fracture. J Hand Surg Am 2015;40:1110–6.
13. Krischak GD, Krasteva A, Schneider F, et al. Physiotherapy after volar plating of wrist fractures is effective using a home exercise program. Arch Phys Med Rehabil 2009;90:537–44.
14. Chung KC, Malay S, Shauver MJ. The relationship between hand therapy and long-term outcomes after distal radius fracture in older adults: Evidence from the randomized wrist and radius injury surgical trial. Plast Reconstr Surg 2019;144(2): 230e–7e.
15. Goudie S, Dixon D, McMillan G, et al. Is use of a psychological workbook associated with improved disabilities of the arm, shoulder and hand scores in patients with distal radius fracture? Clin Orthop Relat Res 2018;476:832–45.
16. Clay FJ, Newstead SV, Watson WL, et al. Bio-psychosocial determinants of persistent pain 6 months after non-life-threatening acute orthopaedic trauma. J Pain 2010;11:420–30.
17. Vranceanu A, Bachoura A, Weening A, et al. Psychological factor predict disability and pain intensity after skeletal trauma. J Bone Joint Surg Am 2014;96: e20.

18. Mehta SP, Macdermid JC, Richardson J, et al. Baseline pain intensity is a predictor of chronic pain in individuals with distal radius fracture. J Orthop Sports Phys Ther 2015;45(2):119–27.

19. British Orthopaedic Association. Best practice for management of distal radius fractures (DRFs). British Society for Surgery of the Hand; 2018. Available at: https://www.bssh.ac.uk/_userfiles/pages/files/professionals/Radius/Blue%20Book%20DRF%20Final%20Document.pdf. Accessed August 1, 2020.

20. Kay S, McMahon M, Stiller K. An advice and exercise program has some benefits over natural recovery after distal radius fracture: a randomised trial. Aust J Physiother 2008;54(4):253–9.

21. Collins DC. Management and rehabilitation of distal radius fractures. Orthop Clin North Am 1993;24(2):365–78.

22. Laseter GF, Carter PR. Management of distal radius fractures. J Hand Ther 1996;9:114–28.

23. Weinstock TB. Management of fractures of the distal radius: therapist's commentary. J Hand Ther 1999;12:99–102.

24. Basso O, Pike JM. The effect of low frequency, long-wave ultrasound therapy on joint mobility and rehabilitation after wrist fracture. J Hand Surg 1998;23-B:136–9.

25. Toomey R, Grief-Schwartz R, Piper MC. Clinical evaluation of the effects of whirlpool on patients with Colles' fractures. Physiother Can 1986;38:280–4.

26. Cheing GL, Wan JW, Kai Lo S. Ice and pulsed electromagnetic field to reduce pain and swelling after distal radius fractures. J Rehabil Med 2005;37(6):372–7.

27. Knygsand-Roenhoej K, Maribo T. A randomized clinical controlled study comparing the effect of modified manual edema mobilization treatment with traditional edema technique in patients with a fracture of the distal radius. J Hand Ther 2011;24(3):184–93.

28. Handoll HH, Elliot J. Rehabilitation for distal radius fractures in adults. Cochrane Database Syst Rev 2015;9:CD003324.

29. Filipova V, Lonzaric D, Papez BJ. Efficacy of combined physical and occupational therapy in patients with conservatively treated distal radius fracture: randomized controlled trial. Wien Klin Wochenschr 2015;127(5):S282–7.

30. Christensen OM, Kunov A, Hansen FF, et al. Occupational therapy and Colles' fractures. Int Orthop 2001;25(1):43–5.

31. Chung KC, Mathews AL. Management of complications of distal radius fractures. Hand Clin 2015;31(2):205–15.

32. Patterson RW, Li Z, Smith BP, et al. Complex regional pain syndrome of the upper extremity. J Hand Surg Am 2011;36(9):1553–62.

33. Li Z, Smith BP, Tuohy C, et al. Complex regional pain syndrome after hand surgery. Hand Clin 2010;26(2):281–9.

34. Jellad A, Salah S, Ben Salah Frih Z. Complex regional pain syndrome type I: incidence and risk factors in patients with fracture of the distal radius. Arch Phys Med Rehabil 2014;95(3):487–92.

35. Jo YH, Kim KW, Lee BG, et al. Incidence of and risk factors for complex regional pain syndrome type 1 after surgery for distal radius fractures: a population-based study. Sci Rep 2019;9(1):4871.

36. Symonette CJ, MacDermid J, Grewal R. Social support contributes to outcomes following distal radius fractures. Rehabil Res Pract 2013;2013:867250.

Complex Regional Pain Syndrome and Distal Radius Fracture
Etiology, Diagnosis, and Treatment

Lauren Kate Dutton, MD, Peter Charles Rhee, DO, MS*

KEYWORDS

- Complex regional pain syndrome • Distal radius fracture • Vitamin C

KEY POINTS

- The incidence of CRPS following distal radius fractures has been reported in the literature as ranging between less than 1% and 51%, which may be secondary to the diagnostic challenges and lack of objective findings associated with this condition.[1–5]
- The diagnosis of CRPS after distal radius fractures remains largely clinical, because imaging modalities have been shown to have poor sensitivity and there are currently no widely available laboratory studies to assist in the diagnosis.
- Risk factors identified for the development of CRPS following distal radius fractures are not uniformly reported but have been identified as older age, female sex, operative treatment of the distal radius fracture, and comorbidities including rheumatoid arthritis and fibromyalgia.[2,3,5–7] The role of psychiatric comorbidities as a potential risk factor for the development of CRPS remains controversial.
- The role of vitamin C in the prevention of CRPS following distal radius fractures remains unclear, with some studies demonstrating a decreased risk of CRPS in patients treated with vitamin C versus placebo and others demonstrating no improvement.[8–14]
- Multiple modalities including physical and occupational therapy, oral pain medications, cognitive-behavioral therapy, sympathetic nerve blocks, and spinal cord stimulation have been proposed for treatment of CRPS. Unfortunately, none of these modalities has consistently demonstrated favorable improvement, and the prognosis for symptomatic relief and return to work is often poor.

INTRODUCTION, DEFINITION, AND BACKGROUND

Complex regional pain syndrome (CRPS) is a chronic pain condition that is characterized by a constellation of signs and symptoms including pain out of proportion to the injury or insult, autonomic dysfunction, trophic changes, and impaired function.[15] Formerly known as reflex sympathetic dystrophy (RSD), the clinical features of this syndrome were first described by French surgeon Ambroise Paré in 1557 and later referred to by Silas Weir Mitchell as "causalgia."[16] In 1929, a committee established by the British Medical Research Council further delineated this latter term with the following description: "spontaneous, diffuse and persistent but subject to exacerbations, excited by stimuli, which do not necessarily produce a physical effect on the limb, and leading to profound changes in the mental state of the patient."[16,17]

Department of Orthopedic Surgery, Mayo Clinic, 200 1st Street Southwest, Rochester, MN 55905, USA
* Corresponding author.
E-mail address: rhee.peter@mayo.edu

Hand Clin 37 (2021) 315–322
https://doi.org/10.1016/j.hcl.2021.02.013
0749-0712/21/© 2021 Elsevier Inc. All rights reserved.

The diagnosis of CRPS was ultimately born out of a Consensus Conference held during the American Pain Society Annual Meeting in 1993, with a proposed definition as follows: "CRPS describes an array of painful conditions that are characterized by a continuing (spontaneous and/or evoked) regional pain that is, seemingly disproportionate in time or degree to the usual course of any known trauma or other lesion. The pain is regional (not in a specific nerve territory or dermatome) and usually has a distal predominance of abnormal sensory, motor, sudomotor, vasomotor, and/or trophic findings. The syndrome shows variable progression over time."[16] In recent years, the diagnostic criteria for CRPS have continued to evolve; the proposed clinical diagnostic criteria for CRPS are described in **Table 1**.

The presence of signs and symptoms indicative of autonomic and inflammatory changes in the particular region where the patient experiences pain is what ultimately distinguishes CRPS as being unique from other pain syndromes.[18] These can include significant allodynia; hyperanalgesia; changes in skin color and temperature; edema; sweating; and decreased range of motion, weakness, and stiffness in the affected region. The onset of these signs and symptoms typically occurs in the wake of peripheral limb trauma, with a resultant exaggeration of the normal post-traumatic inflammatory response.[19]

CRPS has been divided into two distinct subtypes (type I and type II) based on the absence or presence, respectively, of a peripheral nerve injury.[18] CRPS-I, which is more common than type II,[20] was previously referred to as RSD, whereas CRPS-II was previously known as causalgia.[21] Although multiple different inciting events have been linked to the development of CRPS, fractures, and in particular those of the distal radius and ulna, have been cited as the most common antecedent event leading to CRPS type I.[22–24] The application of a tight cast has also been associated with the development of objective signs of CRPS.[24,25] This article provides a comprehensive review of the available literature on the diagnosis and treatment of CRPS in the setting of distal radius fractures.

COMPLEX REGIONAL PAIN SYNDROME AND DISTAL RADIUS FRACTURES: NATURE OF THE PROBLEM

In 1990, Atkins and colleagues[4] reported on the observed features of CRPS or "algodystrophy" in

---

Table 1
Budapest criteria for complex regional pain syndrome

All four of the following criteria must be met:
1. The patient has continuing pain that is disproportionate to any inciting event.
2. The patient demonstrates one sign in at least two of the categories below.
3. The patient reports one symptom in at least three of the categories below.
4. There is no other diagnosis that better explains the patient's presentation.

Category	Signs (Must Display at Least 1 Sign at the Time of Evaluation in 2 or More of the Below Categories)	Symptoms (Must Report at Least 1 Symptom in 3 of the 4 Following Criteria)
Sensory	Evidence of hyperalgesia to pinprick and/or allodynia (to light touch/temperature sensation/deep somatic pressure/joint movement)	Hyperesthesia and/or allodynia
Vasomotor	Evidence of temperature asymmetry (>1°C) and/or: Skin color changes Skin color asymmetry	Temperature asymmetry and/or: Skin color changes Skin color asymmetry
Sudomotor/edema	Evidence of edema and/or: Sweating changes Sweating asymmetry	Edema and/or: Sweating changes Sweating asymmetry
Motor/trophic	Evidence of decreased range of motion and/or: Motor dysfunction (weakness, tremor, dystonia) Trophic changes (hair, nail, skin)	Decreased range of motion and/or: Motor dysfunction (weakness, tremor, dystonia) Trophic changes (hair, nail, skin)

Adapted from Harden RN, Bruehl S, Stanton-Hicks M, et al: Proposed new diagnostic criteria for complex regional pain syndrome. Pain Med 2007;8: pp. 326-331 *and* Neumeister MW, Romanelli MR: Complex regional pain syndrome. Clin Plast Surg 2020 Apr;47(2):305-310.

59 patients treated nonoperatively for[4] Colles fractures. Using a combination of objective measurements and a standardized questionnaire, they found that 9 weeks following distal radius fracture, 24 patients had evidence of vasomotor instability, 23 had tenderness of the fingers, and 23 had lost digital range of motion. Swelling was also noted to be a component of this syndrome. The authors were unable to identify an association between the occurrence of CRPS and the fracture severity, maintenance of fracture reduction, number of manipulations, or age and sex of the patient.

Incidence

Although uncommon in the general population, CRPS has been cited as occurring in 4% to 7% of patients who sustain an extremity fracture or undergo extremity surgery.[18] One population-based study in the Netherlands reported that fractures were the most common precipitating event for CRPS, being cited as the cause of 44% of CRPS cases.[22] A population-based study in Olmsted County, Minnesota, similarly revealed fracture to be the antecedent event leading to CRPS in 46% of cases, likewise making it the most common trigger for this condition.[26] In a study by Sandroni and colleagues,[26] fractures were also associated with the highest rate of resolution of CRPS, including when compared with sprains.

When examining the specific incidence of CRPS following distal radius fractures, the literature reports a wide array of findings ranging from less than 1% to 51%.[1–5] Crijns and colleagues[5] reviewed 59,765 patients treated operatively and nonoperatively for a distal radius fracture between 2012 and 2014 and found that only 114 patients, or 0.19%, were diagnosed with CRPS. Jo and colleagues[2] conducted a population-based study of 172,194 patients treated surgically for distal radius fractures in South Korea between 2007 and 2014 and found the incidence of CRPS-I following distal radius fractures to be low at 0.64%. Moseley and colleagues[1] observed a comparatively higher rate of CRPS in their prospective cohort study of 1549 patients treated conservatively for wrist fractures, noting an incidence of 3.8% of CRPS at 4-month follow-up. Schürmann and colleagues[27] identified an 11% rate of CRPS in their series of 158 patients who sustained distal radius fractures, with an additional 8% of patients being designated as "borderline" given an unclear clinical picture.

Conversely, other authors have demonstrated substantially higher rates of CRPS following distal radius fractures. In their prospective study of 90 patients with distal radius fractures managed with closed reduction and casting, Jellad and

colleagues[6] identified a 32.2% rate of CRPS-I and noted that this was most commonly diagnosed 3 to 4 weeks after cast removal. Demir and colleagues[3] diagnosed 84 of 165 patients with a traumatic injury isolated to the hand or forearm in their study, yielding an incidence of 51%.

Diagnosis

The diagnosis of CRPS frequently remains challenging, particularly given the multiple different diagnostic criteria that have been proposed. Furthermore, the lack of consistent objective findings associated with this condition renders it difficult to definitively diagnose. This is reflected in the wide range of rates of CRPS described in the literature, in population studies, and specifically following distal radius fractures. In a prospective, multicenter cohort study of 596 patients with distal upper or lower extremity fractures, the rate of diagnosis of CRPS ranged from 7.0% (Harden and Bruehl criteria) to 21.3% (criteria of Veldman) to 48.5% (International Association for the Study of Pain criteria) depending on which criteria were used.[28]

On physical examination, the affected limb should be closely observed for skin erythema, pain, warmth, and swelling; over time, however, the injured limb may also become pale and cool.[29] Abnormal posturing or motion of the hand may be present, including intrinsic-minus positioning, dystonia, or tremors.[30] Care should be taken to assess for the presence of a nerve injury, which allows for the distinction between the two subtypes of CRPS.[30] Particularly in the setting of surgically treated distal radius fractures, iatrogenic nerve injuries and neuromas may occur, and thus motor function and the dermatomal distributions of the palmar cutaneous branch of the median nerve, the superficial branch of the radial nerve, and the dorsal ulnar cutaneous nerve should be carefully examined.

Schürmann and colleagues[27] explored the role of various diagnostic imaging modalities including bilateral thermography, plain radiographs, three-phase bone scans, and contrast-enhanced MRIs in 158 patients following distal radius fracture and found that the sensitivity of these modalities was poor (no higher than 45% for any modality) and decreased from the first examination to the final examination at 16 weeks. They did find a high specificity for triple-phase bone scans and MRI at the 8- and 16-week post-trauma intervals (bone scan, 96% and 100%; MRI, 78% and 98%), and a significantly improved specificity of thermography from the second week (50%) to the sixteenth week (89%). These authors concluded that, on account of their poor sensitivity, none of these modalities should be used as screening tests, and that clinical examination remains the gold standard for the diagnosis of CRPS. The findings of this study were confirmed by Gradl and colleagues,[31] who found a low sensitivity and specificity of thermography, and a low sensitivity (33%) but high specificity (91%) for bilateral radiographs. These authors likewise espoused the importance of the clinical examination in the early diagnosis of CRPS-I.

To date, there are no substantiated laboratory values to assist in the work-up of this condition. Recently, Birklein and colleagues[19] reviewed the current evidence for biomarkers in the evaluation of CRPS and reported a potential diagnostic and prognostic role for small noncoding RNAs (microRNAs) to assist in the diagnosis and prognostication of this condition. These authors also noted that given the often evolving nature of this condition, it is unlikely that a single biomarker linked to this condition will be identified.

Predictive and Risk Factors for the Development of Complex Regional Pain Syndrome

Multiple authors have attempted to identify risk factors for the development of CRPS following distal radius fractures to identify and treat this condition in a more expedient fashion.[1–3,5–7,19] Birklein and colleagues[19] noted their observation that patients who experience "an unusually high level of pain during the week after trauma" are at the highest risk for development of CRPS. Moseley and colleagues[1] created a prediction model for the development of CRPS in the setting of nonoperatively treated distal radius and carpal fractures based on four clinical assessments including pain, reaction time, dysynchiria (ie, the provocation of pain in the affected limb while watching the mirror image of the unaffected limb), and swelling, then compared this with a basic assessment of pain intensity on a scale of 1 to 10. They found that this model and the simple pain assessment at 1 week, in accordance with Birklein's observation,[19] correlated strongly with the risk of development of CRPS. Based on their findings, they concluded that a pain score of greater than or equal to five within 1 week of injury in patients treated nonoperatively for distal radius and carpal fractures should be raised as a "red flag" for the future development of CRPS.[1]

Jellad and colleagues[6] identified multiple risk factors for the development of CRPS-I including female sex, trauma of low and medium energy, alteration of physical quality of life as assessed by the Medical Outcomes Study 36-Item Short-Form Health Survey (SF-36), and functional impairment as evaluated by the Patient-Rated Wrist Evaluation scale. They did not find a correlation between CRPS and a history of anxiety and/or depression or radiographic changes. Demir and colleagues[3] found that female patients and those with motor nerve injury were at increased risk for the development of CRPS. Crijns and colleagues[5] identified multiple risk factors for the development of CRPS following distal radius fractures including older age, concomitant distal ulna fracture, and fibromyalgia. Petersen and colleagues[7] reported on the incidence of CRPS following orthopedic treatment of injuries in a Danish population. In their study of 647 patients diagnosed with CRPS, women were five-fold more frequently affected than men, CRPS was reported three times more frequently following surgery as compared with nonoperative treatment, and patients were 2.5 times more likely to have undergone upper extremity surgery as compared with the lower extremity. Jo and colleagues[2] identified multiple risk factors associated with CRPS-I including female sex, rheumatoid arthritis, open reduction, open fracture, and associated ulnar fracture. Advanced age, psychiatric comorbidities, and external fixation were not found to be significantly associated with this syndrome.

Although multiple authors have not found psychiatric comorbidities to be associated with the development of CRPS, Ortiz-Romero and colleagues[32] did find a link between psychiatric history and the onset of CRPS following surgical fixation of distal radius fractures. Worker's compensation, additional fractures, and level of impact were also found to be risk factors in this study.

PREVENTION AND TREATMENT
The Role of Vitamin C in the Prevention of Complex Regional Pain Syndrome

Multiple authors have proposed the administration of vitamin C for the optimization of functional outcome following distal radius fractures and prevention of CRPS.[8] The basis of the rationale for its potential effectiveness is based in part on its efficacy in treating burn patients by attenuating the progression of vascular permeability and reducing microvascular leakage of fluid and proteins, thereby leading to decreased resuscitation fluid requirements and wound edema.[8,10,33,34] Vitamin C has also been shown to accelerate fracture healing in rats via enhanced callus formation[35–37] and to protect skeletal muscle following ischemia-reperfusion injury by reducing tissue edema and neutrophil infiltration.[38,39] Likewise, deficiencies in vitamin C have been shown to result in callus with inferior biomechanical properties.[35] Vitamin

C has also been shown to reduce the incidence developing CRPS after subacromial shoulder surgery when administered prophylactically.[40]

With regard to distal radius fractures in particular, the potential role of vitamin C in decreasing the risk of developing CRPS remains controversial. Zollinger and colleagues[9,10] conducted two randomized controlled trials examining the potential effect of vitamin C on RSD/CRPS in patients with wrist fractures. In their initial trial in 1999,[9] 123 adult patients with 127 distal radius fractures treated with conservative management were randomly allocated to taking vitamin C, 500 mg daily, versus placebo for 50 days. RSD occurred in 7% of the wrists in the vitamin C group as compared with 22% in the placebo group, yielding a relative risk of RSD development of 2.91 in the placebo group (95% confidence interval, 1.02–8.32). Other predictive factors found to have a significant odds ratio included fracture type (AO classification types A and B) and patient complaints of discomfort in the cast in the early stages of immobilization. All patients who developed RSD were female except for 1. Their 2007 study demonstrated similarly encouraging results for the role of vitamin C in CRPS prevention for patients with distal radius fractures. In this study, 416 patients with 427 distal radius fractures were allocated to treatment with placebo versus 200, 500, or 1500 mg of vitamin C daily for 50 days.[10] The overall prevalence of CRPS for patients who were allocated to the vitamin C group was 2.4% as compared with 10.1% in the placebo group ($P = .002$). The two groups with the lowest incidence of CRPS were the 500-mg group and the 1500-mg group at 1.8% and 1.7%, respectively, prompting the authors to recommend a dose of 500 mg daily for 50 days in the setting of distal radius fractures. Similarly to their previous study, early issues with cast wear were found to be predictive of CRPS development, and in this study all patients who developed CRPS were female.

Additional authors have found similarly encouraging benefits of vitamin C in the prevention of CRPS. In their systematic review and meta-analysis of three randomized controlled trials comparing vitamin C 500 mg daily for 50 days starting the day of injury to placebo, Aïm and colleagues found that this dose and duration of vitamin C led to a risk ratio of 0.54 for the development of CRPS-I.[11] Likewise, Meena and colleagues conducted a meta-analysis of four articles and found the incidence of CRPS to be significantly lower in patients treated with vitamin C.[12]

Other studies, however, have failed to reproduce the findings of Zollinger and colleagues Evaniew and colleagues[13] conducted a meta-analysis of three randomized controlled trials comparing vitamin C against placebo for the prevention of CRPS. They found that vitamin C did not reduce the risk of developing CRPS. In their double-blind, randomized controlled trial, Ekrol and colleagues[8] randomized patients who underwent either conservative or surgical treatment of distal radius fractures to either receiving 500 mg of vitamin C or placebo daily for 50 days. In addition to finding that there was no significant effect of vitamin C on the DASH scores throughout the 1-year study period or difference in time to fracture healing, they found a significantly higher rate of CRPS in those patients treated with vitamin C at the 6-week follow-up mark. This association was temporary, because there were no differences found in the rate of CRPS at any other time point. The authors concluded that the administration of vitamin C does not provide any benefit to patients recovering from distal radius fractures.

The 2010 American Academy of Orthopaedic Surgeons clinical practice guidelines for the treatment of distal radius fractures provided a moderate-strength recommendation for the adjuvant treatment of distal radius fractures with vitamin C for the prevention of disproportionate pain.[41] However, the studies by Evaniew (2015) and Ekrol (2014) were published after these clinical practice guidelines and thus would not have been taken into consideration. In 2014, Malay and Chung[14] conducted a literature review to assess the available literature describing the prevention of CRPS with vitamin C after distal radius fracture. They analyzed four articles and a systematic review encompassing these latter articles and concluded that the 2010 American Academy of Orthopaedic Surgeons clinical practice guidelines recommending the use of vitamin C to prevent CRPS after distal radius fractures was valid.

Prognosis and Treatment

Proposed treatment options for CRPS are wide-ranging and have included physical and occupational therapy, oral analgesics, cognitive-behavioral therapy, to invasive options including sympathetic nerve blocks and spinal cord stimulation.[1] Unfortunately, the results of a wide array of treatment modalities for CRPS have not been encouraging, with one study by de Mos and colleagues[42] finding that more than half of CRPS patients evaluated at an average of 5.8 years from the onset of symptoms experienced persistent symptoms, and 16% of these patients reported progressive and worsening symptoms. These findings translated into significant disability, with almost half of patients having a permanent complete or partial job restriction; this included 31% of patients who were completely unable to work and 28% who were able to return to work with adaptations. The findings of this study were more unfavorable than that of Sandroni and colleagues[26] who reported permanent job restrictions in only 11% of patients diagnosed with CRPS.[42]

Bean and colleagues[43] prospectively evaluated patients diagnosed with CRPS-I within 12 weeks of symptomatic onset and again at 6 and 12 months, during which they were evaluated for signs and symptoms of CRPS, pain, depression, anxiety, disability, pain-related fear, stress, and catastrophic thinking using a variety of validated scales. They found that anxiety, pain-related fear, and disability are associated with poorer outcomes in CRPS, indicating potential targets for therapy in the treatment of CRPS.

With the goal of decreasing the exaggerated inflammatory response presumed to be associated with CRPS and stabilizing lysosomal membranes, Atalay and colleagues[44] treated 45 patients diagnosed with CRPS of the upper extremity with a dose of 30 mg of prednisolone that was tapered by 5 mg every 3 days for a total of 3 weeks. After 3 weeks of therapy, these patients demonstrated significant improvements in clinical symptoms and functional and patient-reported outcomes, including visual analog scores (VAS), QuickDASH scores, SF-36 scores, and grip and pinch strength, as compared with baseline. The findings of these authors were reproduced by Bianchi and colleagues,[45] who examined the effects of low-dose oral corticosteroid therapy in the treatment of CRPS in 31 patients and reported significant clinical and functional improvements that persisted up to the 1-year follow-up mark after treatment. They concluded that treatment of CRPS with a short course of low-dose corticosteroids offers a favorable risk-benefit profile. Kalita and colleagues[46] conducted a randomized controlled trial of 60 patients with CRPS following a stroke who were treated with either prednisolone or piroxicam and found that 83.3% of patients treated with prednisolone demonstrated significant improvement versus 16.7% in the piroxicam group. Despite these encouraging findings, a large-scale randomized control trial of the use of corticosteroids in CRPS of the upper extremities following trauma has not been carried out, and this is not a widely used treatment modality despite its potential benefits.[47]

Other proposed oral medications for the treatment of CRPS following hand surgery have included antidepressants, calcium channel blockers, α-blockers, gabapentin, pregabalin, and antiepileptics.[30] Although the relationship between CRPS and psychological comorbidities remains unclear, various counseling therapies have also been proposed.[43]

Several authors have examined the effect of stellate ganglion blockade for the treatment of CRPS-I. Yucel and colleagues[48] performed three stellate ganglion blockades at weekly intervals in 22 patients with CRPS-I, with one group having a shorter symptom onset to treatment interval than the other (mean duration, 17 weeks vs 49.8 weeks). They demonstrated improvement in wrist range of motion and VAS for all patients and relative improvement in the VAS scores of the group with a shorter symptom onset to treatment period, suggesting a role for the early recognition and treatment of CRPS. The results of Ackerman and Zhang[49] for this treatment were less favorable, however, with 40% of patients demonstrating complete relief, 36% reporting partial relief, and 24% describing no relief.

SUMMARY

Because of the relative difficulty of conclusively diagnosing CRPS of the upper extremity following distal radius fractures, the diagnosis of this condition remains elusive, as do its risk factors, incidence, prognosis, and methods of effective treatment. As such, clinicians should have a low threshold to appreciate this condition and become familiar with its clinical diagnostic criteria. A disproportionate amount of pain following either conservative or surgical management of a distal radius fracture should prompt the surgeon to suspect the onset of this condition. The prognosis for this condition remains guarded, and although a wide array of treatment modalities have been described, they may vary in effectiveness.

CLINICS CARE POINTS

- The diagnosis of CRPS after distal radius fractures remains largely clinical based on symptoms and physical examination.

- Risk factors identified for the development of CRPS following distal radius fractures are older age, female sex, operative treatment of the distal radius fracture, and comorbidities including rheumatoid arthritis and fibromyalgia.

- There are conflicting data on the efficacy of vitamin C in the prevention of CRPS following distal radius fractures.

- Many treatment options exist for the management of CRPS, thus highlighting the importance of multimodal and multidisciplinary approach to care.

DISCLOSURE

The authors have nothing to disclose.

REFERENCES

1. Moseley GL, Herbert RD, Parsons T, et al. Intense pain soon after wrist fracture strongly predicts who will develop complex regional pain syndrome: prospective cohort study. J Pain 2014;15(1):16–23.
2. Jo YH, Kim KW, Lee BG, et al. Incidence of and risk factors for complex regional pain syndrome type 1 after surgery for distal radius fractures: a population-based study. Sci Rep 2019;9(1):1–7.
3. Demir SE, Ozaras N, Karamehmetoğlu SS, et al. Risk factors for complex regional pain syndrome in patients with traumatic extremity injury. Ulus Travma Acil Cerrahi Derg 2010;16(2):144–8. Available at: http://www.ncbi.nlm.nih.gov/pubmed/20517769. Accessed May 5, 2020.
4. Atkins RM, Duckworth T, Kanis JA. Features of algodystrophy after Colles' fracture. J Bone Joint Surg Br 1990;72(1):105–10.
5. Crijns TJ, Van Der Gronde BATD, Ring D, et al. Complex regional pain syndrome after distal radius fracture is uncommon and is often associated with fibromyalgia. Clin Orthop Relat Res 2018;476(4): 744–50.
6. Jellad A, Salah S, Ben Salah Frih Z. Complex regional pain syndrome type I: incidence and risk factors in patients with fracture of the distal radius. Arch Phys Med Rehabil 2014;95(3):487–92.
7. Petersen PB, Mikkelsen KL, Lauritzen JB, et al. Risk factors for post-treatment complex regional pain syndrome (CRPS): an analysis of 647 cases of CRPS from the Danish Patient Compensation Association. Pain Pract 2018;18(3):341–9.
8. Ekrol I, Duckworth AD, Ralston SH, et al. The influence of vitamin C on the outcome of distal radial fractures: a double-blind, randomized controlled trial. J Bone Joint Surg Am 2014;96(17):1451–9.
9. Zollinger PE, Tuinebreijer WE, Kreis RW, et al. Effect of vitamin C on frequency of reflex sympathetic dystrophy in wrist fractures: a randomised trial. Lancet 1999;354(9195):2025–8.
10. Zollinger PE, Tuinebreijer WE, Breederveld RS, et al. Can vitamin C prevent complex regional pain syndrome in patients with wrist fractures? A randomized, controlled, multicenter dose-response study. J Bone Joint Surg Am 2007;89(7):1424–31.
11. Aïm F, Klouche S, Frison A, et al. Efficacy of vitamin C in preventing complex regional pain syndrome after wrist fracture: a systematic review and meta-analysis. Orthop Traumatol Surg Res 2017;103(3): 465–70.
12. Meena S, Sharma P, Gangary SK, et al. Role of vitamin C in prevention of complex regional pain syndrome after distal radius fractures: a meta-analysis. Eur J Orthop Surg Traumatol 2015;25(4): 637–41.
13. Evaniew N, Mccarthy C, Kleinlugtenbelt YV, et al. Vitamin C to prevent complex regional pain syndrome in patients with distal radius fractures: a meta-analysis of randomized controlled trials. J Orthop Trauma 2015;29(8):e235–41.
14. Malay S, Chung KC. Testing the validity of preventing chronic regional pain syndrome with vitamin C after distal radius fracture. J Hand Surg Am 2014; 39(11):2251–7.
15. Mathews AL, Chung KC. Management of complications of distal radius fractures. Hand Clin 2015;31(2): 205–15.
16. Stanton-Hicks A, Michael P. CRPS: what's in a name? Taxonomy, epidemiology, neurologic, immune and autoimmune considerations. Reg Anesth Pain Med 2019;44:376–87.
17. Medical Research Council. The diagnosis and treatment of peripheral nerve injuries. Med Res Counc Spec Rep 1920;54:1–59.
18. Bruehl S. Complex regional pain syndrome. BMJ 2015;351.
19. Birklein F, Ajit SK, Goebel A, et al. Complex regional pain syndrome-phenotypic characteristics and potential biomarkers. Nat Rev Neurol 2018;14(5): 272–84.
20. Harden RN, Bruehl S, Perez RSGM, et al. Validation of proposed diagnostic criteria (the "Budapest Criteria") for complex regional pain syndrome. Pain 2010. https://doi.org/10.1016/j.pain.2010.04.030.
21. Shim H, Rose J, Halle S, et al. Complex regional pain syndrome: a narrative review for the practising clinician. Br J Anaesth 2019;123(2):e424–33.
22. de Mos M, de Bruijn AGJ, Huygen FJPM, et al. The incidence of complex regional pain syndrome: a population-based study. Pain 2007;129(1–2):12–20.
23. Bickerstaff DR, Kanis JA. Algodystrophy: an under-recognized complication of minor trauma. Rheumatology 1994. https://doi.org/10.1093/rheumatology/33.3.240.
24. Neumeister MW, Romanelli MR. Complex regional pain syndrome. Clin Plast Surg 2020. https://doi.org/10.1016/j.cps.2019.12.009.
25. Field J, Protheroe DL, Atkins RM. Algodystrophy: after Colles fractures is associated with secondary tightness of casts. J Bone Joint Surg Br 1994. https://doi.org/10.1302/0301-620x.76b6.7983115.
26. Sandroni P, Benrud-Larson LM, McClelland RL, et al. Complex regional pain syndrome type I: incidence and prevalence in Olmsted county, a population-based study. Pain 2003;103(1–2):199–207.
27. Schürmann M, Zaspel J, Löhr P, et al. Imaging in early posttraumatic complex regional pain syndrome: a comparison of diagnostic methods. Clin J Pain 2007;23(5):449–57.

28. Beerthuizen A, Stronks DL, Van'T Spijker A, et al. Demographic and medical parameters in the development of complex regional pain syndrome type 1 (CRPS1): prospective study on 596 patients with a fracture. Pain 2012;153(6):1187–92.

29. Ratti C, Nordio A, Resmini G, et al. Post-traumatic complex regional pain syndrome: clinical features and epidemiology. Clin Cases Miner Bone Metab 2015;12(Suppl 1):11.

30. Li Z, Smith BP, Tuohy C, et al. Complex regional pain syndrome after hand surgery. Hand Clin 2010. https://doi.org/10.1016/j.hcl.2009.11.001.

31. Gradl G, Steinborn M, Wizgall I, et al. Acute CRPS I (Morbus Sudeck) following distal radial fractures - methods for early diagnosis. Zentralbl Chir 2003. https://doi.org/10.1055/s-2003-44851.

32. Ortiz-Romero J, Bermudez-Soto I, Torres-González R, et al. Factors associated with complex regional pain syndrome in surgically treated distal radius fracture. Acta Ortop Bras 2017;25(5):194–6.

33. Tanaka H, Matsuda T, Miyagantani Y, et al. Reduction of resuscitation fluid volumes in severely burned patients using ascorbic acid administration: a randomized, prospective study. Arch Surg 2000; 135(3):326–31.

34. Matsuda T, Tanaka H, Shimazaki S, et al. High-dose vitamin C therapy for extensive deep dermal burns. Burns 1992;18(2):127–31.

35. Alcantara-Martos T, Delgado-Martinez AD, Vega MV, et al. Effect of vitamin C on fracture healing in elderly osteogenic disorder Shionogi rats. J Bone Joint Surg Br 2007;89(3):402–7.

36. Sarisözen B, Durak K, Dinçer G, et al. The effects of vitamins E and C on fracture healing in rats. J Int Med Res 2002;30(3):309–13.

37. Yilmaz C, Erdemli E, Selek H, et al. The contribution of vitamin C to healing of experimental fractures. Arch Orthop Trauma Surg 2001;121(7):426–8.

38. Kearns SR, Moneley D, Murray P, et al. Oral vitamin C attenuates acute ischaemia-reperfusion injury in skeletal muscle. J Bone Joint Surg Br 2001;83(8): 1202–6.

39. Kearns SR, Daly AF, Sheehan K, et al. Oral vitamin C reduces the injury to skeletal muscle caused by compartment syndrome. J Bone Joint Surg Br 2004;86(6):906–11.

40. Laumonerie P, Martel M, Tibbo ME, et al. Influence of vitamin C on the incidence of CRPS-I after subacromial shoulder surgery. Eur J Orthop Surg Traumatol 2020;30(2):221–6.

41. Lichtman DM, Bindra RR, Boyer MI, et al. Treatment of distal radius fractures. J Am Acad Orthop Surg 2010. https://doi.org/10.5435/00124635-201003000-00007.

42. De Mos M, Huygen FJPM, Van Der Hoeven-Borgman M, et al. Outcome of the complex regional pain syndrome. Clin J Pain 2009;25(7):590–7.

43. Bean DJ, Johnson MH, Heiss-Dunlop W, et al. Do psychological factors influence recovery from complex regional pain syndrome type 1? A prospective study. Pain 2015;156(11):2310–8.

44. Atalay NS, Ercidogan O, Akkaya N, et al. Prednisolone in complex regional pain syndrome. Pain Physician; 2014.

45. Bianchi C, Rossi S, Turi S, et al. Long-term functional outcome measures in corticosteroid-treated complex regional pain syndrome. Eura Medicophys 2006;42(2):103–11.

46. Kalita J, Vajpayee A, Misra UK. Comparison of prednisolone with piroxicam in complex regional pain syndrome following stroke: a randomized controlled trial. QJM 2006. https://doi.org/10.1093/qjmed/hcl004.

47. Winston P. Early treatment of acute complex regional pain syndrome after fracture or injury with prednisone: Why is there a failure to treat? A case series. Pain Res Manag 2016. https://doi.org/10.1155/2016/7019196.

48. Yucel I, Demiraran Y, Ozturan K, et al. Complex regional pain syndrome type I: efficacy of stellate ganglion blockade. J Orthop Traumatol 2009;10(4):179–83.

49. Ackerman WE, Zhang JM. Efficacy of stellate ganglion blockade for the management of type 1 complex regional pain syndrome. South Med J 2006; 99(10):1084–8.

Moving?

Make sure your subscription moves with you!

To notify us of your new address, find your **Clinics Account Number** (located on your mailing label above your name), and contact customer service at:

Email: journalscustomerservice-usa@elsevier.com

800-654-2452 (subscribers in the U.S. & Canada)
314-447-8871 (subscribers outside of the U.S. & Canada)

Fax number: 314-447-8029

Elsevier Health Sciences Division
Subscription Customer Service
3251 Riverport Lane
Maryland Heights, MO 63043

ELSEVIER

Printed and bound by CPI Group (UK) Ltd, Croydon, CR0 4YY

08/05/2025

01864704-0015